Community Mental Health Nursing

The Practitioner's Point of View

The opinions expressed in this volume are the authors' and not necessarily those of the advisory committee for the community mental health nursing conference of ANA.

This project was supported by USPHS Training Grant No.1 T14 MH12119–01 from the National Institute of Mental Health.

Community Mental Health Nursing
The Practitioner's Point of View

Edited by Elaine Goldman, R.N., M.S.

APPLETON-CENTURY-CROFTS
EDUCATIONAL DIVISION/MEREDITH CORPORATION
New York

PRINTED IN THE UNITED STATES OF AMERICA

390-37027-4

Advisory Committee

Chairman: Mrs. Rachel A. Robinson, M.A., R.N.
Assistant Professor of Nursing, Yale University School of Nursing, 310 Cedar Street, New Haven, Connecticut

Mrs. Ruth V. Lewis, M.A., R.N.
Director of Program Development & Evaluation, Greater Kansas City Mental Health Foundation, 600 East 22nd Street, Kansas City, Missouri

C. Elizabeth Madore, M.A., R.N.
Associate Professor of Nursing, Arizona State University, College of Nursing, Tempe, Arizona

Janice E. Ruffin, M.S., R.N.
Supervisor-Clinician, Inpatient Psychiatry, Soundview-Throgs Neck Community, Mental Health Center, 2527 Glebe Avenue, Bronx, New York

Mrs. Ruth Q. Seigler, B.S., R.N.
Chief Nurse, Columbia Area Mental Health Center, 2550 Colonial Drive, Columbia, South Carolina

Speakers

Sarah Helen Carlton, M.N., R.N.
Psychiatric Nursing Specialist, Bay County Guidance Clinic, 615 North MacArthur Avenue, Panama City, Florida

Toni M. Francis, M.A., R.N.
Mental Health Worker, Arthur Capper Clinic, 1011 7th Street, S. E., Washington, D. C.

Nancy H. French, M.S., R.N.
Associate Director of Nursing, Connecticut Mental Health Center, 34 Park Street, New Haven, Connecticut; and Assistant Professor, Yale University School of Nursing

Mrs. Sharon Gedan, M.S., R.N.
Clinical Specialist, Psychiatric Nursing, The Straub Clinic, Department of Psychiatry, 888 South King Street, Honolulu, Hawaii

Judith Anne Martois, M.S., R.N.
Public Health Nursing Consultant, San Gabriel Valley Mental Health Service, 330 East Live Oak, Arcadia, California

Mr. Norman Morse, M.A., R.N.
Instructor, Division of Nurse Education, New York University, Washington Square, New York, New York

Anita L. Narciso, M.S., R.N.
Community Mental Health Liaison Nurse, Baltimore City Health Department, American Building, Baltimore & South Street, Baltimore, Maryland

Justina D. Neufeld, B.S., R.N.
Community Mental Health Center Nurse, Prairie View Community Mental Health Center, P.O. Box 467, Newton, Kansas

Mrs. Judith Betz Proctor, R.N.
Head Nurse, Drug Dependence Unit, Connecticut Mental Health Center, 104-106 Park Street, New Haven, Connecticut

Mrs. Janelle Smith Ramsburg, M.S.W., R.N. Director, Nursing Education, Western Missouri Mental Health Center, 600 East 22nd Street, Kansas City, Missouri

Mrs. Hilda Richards, Ed.M., R.N.
Assistant Chief, Harlem Rehabilitation Center, 121 West 128 Street, New York, New York

Margene Tower, M.S., R.N.
Assistant Director of Nursing, Denver General Hospital, Division of Psychiatry, 6th & Cherokee, Denver, Colorado

Participants

Mrs. Eva Anderson, B.S., R.N.
Mental Health Consultant, Northwestern Mental Health Center, Crookston, Minnesota

Ellen A. Andruzzi, M.S., R.N.
Chief, Division of Mental Health Nursing, Department of Public Health, District of Columbia, 801 North Capitol St., N.E.–Room 631, Washington, D. C.

Mrs. Lois I. Batton, R.N.
Coordinator, Halifax County Mental Health Center, P.O. Box 577, Roanoke Rapids, North Carolina

Mrs. Esther M. Bigelow, M.S., R.N.
Psychiatric Nursing Coordinator, Hennepin County Mental Health Center, 5th & Portland, Minneapolis, Minnesota

Cherryl L. Blakeway, M.P.N., R.N.
Assistant Director of Nursing Service, Creighton Memorial St. Joseph Hospital, 2305-10th Street, Omaha, Nebraska

Mrs. Joye C. Bradley, M.N., R.N.
Principal Nurse Consultant, Georgia Department of Public Health, Division of Mental Health, 47 Trinity Avenue, Atlanta, Georgia

Mrs. Mary R. Cantrell, M.S., R.N.
Associate Chief, Nursing Service for Education, Veterans Administration Hospital, Waco, Texas

Mrs. Frances R. Carbone, R.N.
Psychiatric Nurse, Northern Wyoming Mental Health Center, P.O. Box 4098, Sheridan, Wyoming

Mrs. Elizabeth Carter, M.S., R.N.
Assistant Professor, School of Nursing, Adelphi University, Garden City, New York

Mrs. Linda Copeland, B.S., R.N.
Supervisor of Nursing, Hahnemann Community Mental Health Center, In-Patient and Day Hospital, 314 No. Broad Street, Philadelphia, Pennsylvania

Rose Marie Davidites, M.A., R.N.
Director, Nursing Service, Maimonides Community Mental Health Center, 1048 48th Street, Brooklyn, New York

Richard E. Drake, M.S., R.N.
Director, Division of Nursing, Central Utah Community Mental Health Center, 160 East Center, Provo, Utah

Mrs. Rhetaugh Graves Dumas, M.S.N., R.N. Director of Nursing, Connecticut Mental Health Center, 34 Park Street, New Haven, Connecticut; and Associate Professor, Yale University, School of Nursing, New Haven, Connecticut

Fernando A. Duran, M.S., R.N.
Coordinator of Mental Health Nursing, Northeast Kingdom Mental Health Services, 90 Main Street, Box 245, Newport, Vermont

Mrs. Nancy B. Fasano, M.S.N., R.N.
Acting Director of Nursing, St. Lawrence Community Mental Health Center, 1201 West Oakland Avenue, Lansing, Michigan

Cathleen Getty, M.S., R.N.
Associate Professor, School of Nursing, State University of New York at Buffalo, Health Sciences Building, Buffalo, New York; and Consultant, Erie County Suicide Prevention and Crisis Center, 560 Main Street, Buffalo, New York

Priscilla B. Gretsch, M.S., R.N.
Clinical Specialist, Psychiatric Nursing, Jefferson County Mental Health Center, Inc., 260 S. Kipling, Lakewood, Colorado

Mrs. Marie J. Groth, B.S.N., R.N.
Nurse Specialist, Mental Health, Linn County Mental Health Clinic, Court House Annex, Albany, Oregon

Mrs. Margaret A. Hardin, M.A., R.N.
Director of Nursing, Maricopa County General Hospital, 3435 W. Durango, Phoenix, Arizona

Mrs. Catherine Neighbor Harris, M.S., R.N. Public Health Nursing Consultant, Bernalillo County Community Mental Health Center, 2600 Marble N.E., Albuquerque, New Mexico; and Assistant Professor of Psychiatry, Department of Psychiatry, University of New Mexico School of Medicine

Mary C. Henderson, M.S., R.N.
Mental Health Nurse, Montgomery Area Mental Health Center, 345 So. Ripley St., Montgomery, Alabama

Lydia Hill, M.S., R.N.
Coordinator, Division of Consultation and Education, Central State Community Mental Health Center, Villa & Alameda St., Box 151, Norman, Oklahoma

Mrs. Janice Hitchcock, M.S., R.N.
Lecturer, Community Mental Health Nursing, University of California, San Francisco Medical Center, 1483 4th Avenue, San Francisco, California

Mrs. Sharon Janzen, B.S.N., R.N.
Psychiatric Nursing Consultant, Marquette-Alger-Delta Community Mental Health Center, Altamont & Fisher, Marquette, Michigan

Mrs. Margaret N. Johnson, R.N.
Psychiatric Nurse, Appalachian Comprehensive Care Center, 1539 Central Ave.–P.O. Box 790, Ashland, Kentucky

Evelyn J. Kennedy, M.A., R.N.
Assistant Professor, Meharry Medical College, 1005 18th Avenue, North, Nashville, Tennessee

A. Naomi Kennedy, M.A., R.N.
Regional Mental Health Nurse Consultant, National Institute of Mental Health, DHEW–Region III, 220 7th N.E., Charlottesville, Virginia

Linda Harrison Laws, B.S., R.N.
Head Nurse (Mental Health Nurse II), W. H. Trentman Mental Health Center, 3008 New Bern Avenue, Raleigh, North Carolina

Mrs. Evelyn M. McElroy, M.S., R.N.
Doctoral candidate, University of Maryland School of Nursing, School of Medicine, Baltimore, Maryland; Clinical Specialist in Inner-City Community Mental Health Program

Mrs. Sandra L. Matteson, M.S., R.N.
Nurse Clinician, Counseling Service, 302 Wooster, Marietta, Ohio; and Psychiatric Nursing Consultant, State of Ohio Mental Health & Retardation Board, 648, 13 West Washington Street, Athens, Ohio

Nancy Mayes, B.S., R.N.
Assistant in Instruction, Psychiatric Nursing, Cornell University–New York Hospital School of Nursing, 1320 York Avenue, New York, New York

Mrs. Donna Miller, M.S., R.N.
Director of Psychiatric Nursing, Marion County Community Mental Health Center and Psychiatry Department of Marion County General Hospital, 960 Locke Street, Indianapolis, Indiana

Mrs. Ruth S. Miller, M.P.H., R.N.
Mental Health Consultant, St. Josephs Hospital and St. Josephs Hospital School of Nursing, Hancock, Michigan

Judith Moore, M.S., R.N.
Instructor, Graduate Program in Advanced Psychiatric Nursing, Rutgers University, College of Nursing, 91 Halsey Street, Newark, New Jersey

Mrs. Mabel Morris, M.A., R.N.
Chief Nurse, Temple University Community Mental Health Center, 1424 W. Ontario Street, Philadelphia, Pennsylvania

Mrs. Mary Ann Muranko, M.S., R.N.
Community-Hospital Liaison Nurse, Nursing Department, Children's Psychiatric Hospital, University of Michigan, Ann Arbor, Michigan

Cornelius E. Neufeld, M.S., R.N.
Director of Mental Health Nursing, Western Missouri Mental Health Center, 600 East 22nd Street, Kansas City, Missouri

Phyllis Parnes, D.N.Sc., R.N.
Clinical Specialist, Connecticut Mental Health Center, 34 Park Street, New Haven, Connecticut; and Instructor, Yale University School of Nursing, New Haven, Connecticut

Mrs. Elizabeth M. Patterson, B.S., R.N.
Program Director, Hospital Staff Development Grant for Nursing Inservice Education, Terrell State Hospital, Box 70, Terrell, Texas

Mrs. Norma Schapera, M.S., R.N.
Assistant Director of Nursing, Hamilton County Diagnostic Clinics, 295 Erkenbrecher Avenue, Cincinnati, Ohio

Kathryn A. Schlichtmann, M.A., R.N.
Community Nurse Specialist, Olympic Center for Mental Health and Mental Retardation, P.O. Box 4099, Wycoff Station, Bremerton, Washington

Sister Sheila Lyne, M.S., R.N.
Chief Nurse Therapist, Community Mental Health Center of Scott County, 2322 Marquette, Davenport, Iowa; and Assistant Professor, University of Iowa, College of Nursing, Iowa City, Iowa

Sister Ann McCormack, M.S., R.N.
Supervisor, De Paul Hospital, New Orleans, Louisiana

Jonna Kate Smith, M.S., R.N.
Mental Health Community Nurse II, Pilsen Outpost of the Community Mental Health Program of Westside Medical Center, 1642 So. Blue Island, Chicago, Illinois

M. Anita Stoddard, B.S., R.N.
Mental Health Nurse, Columbia Area Mental Health Center, 2550 Colonial Drive, Columbia, South Carolina

Barbara E. Teague, M.S., R.N.
Director of Nurses, Dr. Harry C. Solomon Mental Health Center, 391 Varnum Avenue, Lowell, Massachusetts

Phyllis Elizabeth Wentz, R.N.
Assistant Professor, Psychiatric Nursing-Community Mental Health, University of North Dakota, College of Nursing, Grand Forks, North Dakota

Concha Yenoukian, R.N.
Psychiatric Area Supervisor, Sacramento Medical Center, 2315 Stockton Blvd., Sacramento, California

Mrs. Rothlyn Zahourek, M.S., R.N.
Psychiatric Research Nurse: Clinical Specialist, Department of Health and Hospitals, Division of Psychiatric Services, Denver General Hospital, 201 West 6th Avenue, Denver, Colorado

Guests

Herbert J. Butler, Ed.D., R.N.
Nurse Consultant, Community Mental Health Centers, Division, Mental Health Services Development Branch, National Institute of Mental Health, 5454 Wisconsin Avenue, Chevy Chase, Maryland

Alice Clarke, M.A., R.N.
Editor, Perspectives in Psychiatric Care, 194B Kinderkamack Road, Park Ridge, New Jersey

Gertrude Johannsen, M.Ed.
Consultant, Division of Community Services, National League for Nursing, 10 Columbus Circle, New York, New York

Winifred Maher, M.S.N.E., R.N.
Acting Chief, Psychiatric Nursing, Training Branch, Division of Manpower & Training Programs, National Institute of Mental Health, 5454 Wisconsin Avenue, Chevy Chase, Maryland

Mrs. Dorothy Nayer, M.A., R.N.
Associate Editor, American Journal of Nursing, 10 Columbus Circle, New York, New York

Mrs. Jeannette Nehren, M.S., R.N.
Chief, Nursing & Related Therapeutic Personnel Section, Continuing Education Branch, Manpower Training, National Institute of Mental Health, 5454 Wisconsin Avenue, Chevy Chase, Maryland

Alice Robinson, M.S., R.N.,
Editor, Nursing Outlook, 10 Columbus Circle, New York, New York

Frank Tosiello, Ed.D., R.N.
Nursing Consultant, Department of Mental Hygiene, Office of Manpower and Training, 44 Holland Avenue, Albany, New York

Frances Williams, M.S., R.N.
Nurse Consultant, Department of Health, Education & Welfare, Region II, 26 Federal Plaza, New York, New York

ANA Staff

Mrs. Barbara Allen Davis, M.S., R.N.
Program Coordinator, Division on Psychiatric and Mental Health Nursing Practice

Mrs. Kathryn Wheeler
Assistant Director, Public Relations Department

Preface

In the past, nursing practice has sporadically included social and political activities, and individual nurses have been advocates for their patients' rights. However, such expanded practice has not been examined by the profession as a whole until the Community Mental Health Centers Act of 1963 brought into clear focus the problems and challenges of a society in crisis. With the establishment of community-based mental health programs, a system of mental health and psychiatric services was provided which would enable clients to continue to function as members of the community. The philosophical base thus established required a different approach to the delivery of mental health-psychiatric services. The subsequent rapid development of these programs and the concomitant need for skilled manpower exerted pressure on the nursing profession to educate and supply nurse practitioners for a variety of mental health programs.

Psychiatric nursing practitioners and educators, using standards of practice established by the American Nurses' Association, sought guidance from the professional organization in planning and developing programs, initiating processes, and identifying nursing roles in community mental health. Over the years, the Psychiatric Nursing Conference Group and later the Division on Psychiatric-Mental Health Nursing Practice has been concerned with the increasing need and demand for mental health services and personnel. The Division's executive committee sought funds from the Division of Mental Health Services Development Branch of the National Institute of Mental Health to enable the ANA to carry out its plans for sponsoring a national conference on community mental health nursing practice. Community mental health nursing practitioners, selected from all over the United States, convened in New York City on February 25-27, 1970 to share their broad range of experiences, ideas, and opinions. The ultimate purpose of the conference was to describe the nature and scope of community mental health nursing practice and problems, and to gain knowledge of new and innovative forms of practice. The papers and discussions of the conference plus three theoretical papers on subjects deemed necessary to the practice of community mental health nursing will be found in this book.

The book is really about people, primarily community mental health nurses, and their ability to make meaningful human contacts. Such contacts between nurses and clients have led to collaborative endeavors to enable clients to cope with the pathogenic social conditions which have thwarted their growth. The speakers and other conferees told of being in touch with people's fear, isolation, frustration, anger, and pain; they talked about dealing with issues which affect people deeply: sex, racism, deprivation, power, and politics; they stressed the fact that the goal of community mental health programs is to provide service that is relevant to the needs of the people; and they agreed that the encounter with the client and his social system encourages a mutual learning process whereby the client is assisted in identifying his needs, making them known, and solving his problems, thus gaining a sense of powerfulness.

Conference Postulates

For nursing practice to be relevant to the needs of clients and communities, the conferees advanced the following premises:

1. The community mental health nurse bases her concept of clients' needs on priorities established by the client.
2. Community mental health nursing is not limited solely to dealing with psychiatric problems.
3. The final responsibility for solving his problems rests with the client. The community mental health nurse is the facilitator, working collaboratively with clients, other professionals, paraprofessionals, and members of the community.
4. The community mental health nurse has a responsibility to become involved with social issues and to participate in social action and subsequent social change in order to institute and implement preventive programs relevant to individuals, families, and the community.
5. If the community mental health nurse is to be an effective change agent, she should possess theoretical knowledge and understanding of social systems, power, and change.
6. The community mental health nurse must develop a carefully planned program which includes sensitivity to the vested interests and feelings of others.

Problems Encountered

The above postulates are deceptively simple. Although many community mental health programs purport to encourage their use, actual practice falls far short of the rhetoric. A few of the complex problems community mental health nurses encounter are summarized here:

1. Establishing relationships with: (a) the larger nursing system; (b) members of the black and Puerto Rican communities; (c) other professionals, paraprofessionals, and "new careerists."
2. Recognizing, utilizing, and sharing power.
3. Intervening with the social and political structure in the mental health facility, the community, municipality, state and federal systems.

A recurring theme which emerged at the conference was that nurses must develop competence and power in order to cope with the complexities facing all community mental health workers. Nurses must avoid rationalizing their inadequacy by blaming it on forces beyond their control.

The experiences, ideas, and feelings expressed during the conference represent some of the viewpoints needed by community mental health practitioners, employers, and educators in order to provide a basis for further clarification and conceptualization of the philosophy and practice of community mental health nursing. In addition, the concepts presented in this book should interest and influence psychiatric nursing conference groups within state and district nurses associations to hold similar conference-workshops and to stimulate nursing research.

It is our hope that the book will acquaint people with an understanding of the nature, excitement, and significance of the nurse's role in community mental health programs. It could serve as a recruitment device to draw nurses into community mental health nursing and attract energetic young people into the nursing profession who will seek constructive involvement in the current social crisis.

The first four sections correspond to the four major topics selected for the conference. These topics are not only interrelated but are inseparable in practice. Similar themes and issues seemed to recur in relation to each topic, despite the diversity of content and the heterogeneity of the speakers. The papers and related discussions involve the reader in the immediacy of universal human experience. Conferees reported that community mental health nurses, as well as other community health personnel, learn about social systems, power, and change primarily through the work situation, which often is too little and too late. Chapters in Part Two present theoretical explorations considered necessary for the assessment and maintenance of, or intervention in, the various interacting mental health processes and systems. Selected experts were asked to write these chapters following the conference.

Part Three represents the planning, implementation, and outcome of the conference. It includes the grant proposal, objectives and design of the conference, a glossary, an overview of content and process, recommendations and an evaluation of the conference, and an annotated bibliography submitted by the conferees.

About the Editor

Elaine Goldman has worked in staff positions as a visiting nurse in the community and as a psychiatric nurse in a therapeutic milieu treatment hospital. Mrs. Goldman received her Master's degree in psychiatric nursing from Adelphi University, Garden City, New York. She was Director of the Mental Health Project at the Skidmore College Department of Nursing.

The production of this book developed as a result of her role as Director of this ANA project, the first Conference on Community Mental Health Nursing.

Currently, Mrs. Goldman is an assistant professor in the Adelphi University School of Nursing Continuing Education Project. She is involved in human relations training via workshops, short courses, and sensitivity training programs.

She is a member of the American Nurses' Association, National League for Nursing, and the American Society for Training and Development.

Message From The President

This is an auspicious time for the ANA through this Conference on Community Mental Health Nursing to lend the voice of nurses and organized nursing to the call for solution of the problems of a "Society in Crisis."

Poverty, pollution, crime, race problems, disintegration of our cities, war, violence, drug abuse, a near bankrupt educational system, population growth—these and other glaring social problems all impinge upon health. Nurses, along with other professionals and all other socially-minded citizens, must speak to these problems and help to solve them. For mental health is an outcome of opportunities to live in environments and to participate in interpersonal systems that enhance development of one's capacities and that promote joyous use of one's competencies.

The World Health Organization definition of health as not merely the absence of disease but a sense of well-being and full self-development is being taken seriously. There is increasing concern about life and the quality of living, and health as an essential ingredient for all people. In realizing these changing values, nurses have a vital role to play.

Nursing as a profession is more than tending the sick and includes services toward prevention of illness and community involvement. Indeed, it was nurses who gave initial impetus to developing prenatal care, baby welfare stations, health teaching, especially among the poor, and many such activities including community mental health that underlie the present, social interest in improving the quality of living of all people of the world.

Community mental health nurses, through direct and indirect nursing services have played and will continue to play a significant role in shifting the focus to self-fulfillment and self-determination for all individuals in society. But more than this is needed to meet the broadening interests in health of our citizens. Nurses must opt also for nurse power—by uniting together and pooling their collective strengths and resources so that nurses as a group can speak vigorously and act effectively in society. That is what ANA is all about—a collectivity of nurses that asserts nurse power, that voices the united views of nurses on health matters, and that sees to it that society takes these united views into account and implements them.

This publication provides a report of one conference for selected nurses held under the auspices of ANA, in which the held views of nurses addressed to questions and issues in mental health work are presented. In sharing the nature of their work and their opinions with others, a basis for further dialogue on these matters is made available. It is in this way—discussion, formulation, reaction and further discussion—that clarification of the phenomena of mental health and nursing practice occurs. There is much for all disciplines still to learn about the field of mental health work. In this continuing process this contribution of expert nurses working in mental health facilities is worthy of attention.

Hildegard E. Peplau, R.N., Ed.D.
President
American Nurses' Association

Contents

PART ONE–CURRENT INNOVATIONS IN COMMUNITY MENTAL HEALTH NURSING PRACTICE

Part One
Current Innovations
In Community
Mental Health
Nursing Practice

Treatment Modalities

There is a great need for relevant mental health services among the disadvantaged for whom traditional patterns of psychiatry and the delivery of services are not only inadequate but in many cases inappropriate. The task of mental health workers is to develop programs and methods based on an ideology that is compatible and also responsive to the value systems and life styles of clients. In some urban areas, clients believe that relevant health service is their right and they are actively involved in bringing about change in mental health services. In other areas, mental health workers are helping clients to make demands for relevant service.

Personnel in the field of mental health have been experiencing a shift to new programs and new services since 1963 but the position of nursing personnel remains unclear. Despite the undefined role and the lack of sufficient numbers of prepared practitioners, the nursing profession must take some action in order to increase, through effective practice, the relevance of mental health nursing services.

In describing the nurse's involvement in treatment modalities, conferees found it necessary to explore the expanding role and function of nurses in community mental health concomitantly. What is the role, function, and power of the community mental health nurse? The answer to that question depends on the many variables involved in the nurse's position, education, clinical and life experience, personal ability and stature; the philosophy, organization, and administration of the agency, and the services offered in the agency; the characteristics of the client and the community being served; the nurse's view of psychiatric-mental health care in general, and psychiatric-mental health nursing in particular. These variables change and the nurse's role, function, and power change accordingly.

Despite the efforts of a few conferees to specify what nurses can or cannot do, the majority held such efforts to be a detriment. "Don't box us in," they said. There was consensus that the nurse's role is an evolving one which permits fluidity and flexibility in response to the needs of clients and the characteristics of the community. This point of view affords the nurse the opportunity to develop skills in addition to those she has practiced as a result of her educational preparation.

Conferees reported how they had participated innovatively in various treatment modalities in response to the shifting needs of their clients. For example, mobility was provided by visits to individuals, families, community groups, and by bringing mobile crisis and aftercare units to the local communities. They reported that community mental health nurses are involved in a variety of therapies such as individual, group, and family psychotherapy; milieu, reality, behavior, and play therapies; psychodrama, sensitivity encounter, and mini marathon activities; preventive and aftercare activity groups. They reported active involvement in community organizations and in confrontation and protest activities; in the initiation and coordination of community resource councils; in the provision of liaison services to general hospitals, psychiatric hospitals, and related agencies. Workers' accessibility was made possible by decentralized clinics, 24-hour, seven-day week services, drop-in clinics, and lunch-hour, evening, and weekend groups. Manpower extension was made possible by offering and giving consultation to nursing personnel in public health agencies, general hospitals, state hospitals, and geriatric facilities, school principals, teachers, police, clergy, community leaders, and volunteers in the health fields.

Conferees agreed that it is no longer sufficient for the nurse to be concerned solely with the health and welfare of the patient who actively seeks help. Those who most frequently need help do not look for it. Nurses must pursue those individuals not being cared for, those patients for whom, in many cases, no one is caring. Some conferees reported that "persistence and pursuit" has emerged as a high priority policy in community mental health nursing in rural and urban areas; others reported a different policy in which clients are required to seek out mental health service. However, conferees agreed that one of the major goals in their work was to enable the client to become self-determining and more powerful.

Nurses are trying to offer qualitative and quantitative services to individuals and communities, giving to recipients at the same time realistic opportunities to decide what the nature of the services should be. Conferees reported incidents of successful collaboration (as well as struggles) with members of other systems such as nursing organizations, hospital and public health nursing personnel, individuals and groups of other professional disciplines, paraprofessionals, clients, ex-clients, volunteers, and members of mental health boards and councils.

Some examples of the "struggles" included: (1) negotiating with a real estate agent or landlord to provide a store for use as a mental health facility; and (2) conveying the nature of the mental health program to a lay person or a lay group who perceives clients as "crazy nuts." One conferee summed up her experience: "You win a few—you lose a few; you sometimes need to pull back, augment your forces, negotiate for power, and re-enter, but always go back."

The conferees differed in their perceptions of their respective roles which included therapist, team leader, consultant, and liaison worker. However, they agreed on their major concern and purpose for being: how best to determine the clients' and community's needs and find the most expedient way to provide the necessary services. With this purpose in mind, they vigorously contested what they considered to be "ripples of change without the accompanying and necessary underlying ideological changes." They believed that much of their work had creative qualities, but argued that they themselves were still too pathology-oriented. The question arose as to whether mental health center staff should continue to care for the patient who is sick or, instead, focus on prevention. They concluded that both fall within the province of community mental health nursing. Conferees expressed need for more knowledge of social systems theory such as concepts of power and change, in order to direct their energies towards appropriate changes for the benefit of the whole community and society.

Nurses are oriented traditionally to the interrelationship of physiological, psychological, and sociological phenomena. The nurse, more than other mental health workers, is alert to physiological processes, and is aware of body image, and the nurse is sensitive to the patient's perception of his image, his moods, and his feelings. Nurses were described as having proven themselves to be flexible, accessible, practical, and able to focus on solving immediate problems. Certainly in working with the disadvantaged client, the above characteristics serve the nurse well.

The definition of nursing or the identification of nursing roles, functions, and activities is an unending process, difficult at best and often controversial in nursing groups as well as related disciplines. To describe nursing practice in a complex field like community mental health is fraught with the danger of oversimplification. In the following report, the facts and opinions presented by both speakers and discussants is an attempt to share their experiences as community mental health nursing practitioners.

Community Mental Health Nurses
Question "Care, Cure and Coordination"

ROTHLYN ZAHOUREK, R.N., M.S.
MARGENE TOWER, R.N., M.S.

The role of the nurse can no longer be described by a single word or even a number of words. As nurses move into community mental health centers the terms "care," "cure," and "coordination" become less and less relevant. These terms, proposed by the American Nurses' Association's Position Paper in 1965, have served as a valuable basis for discussion, but are now practically obsolete for defining the role of the nurse.[1] Rather than promoting a professional image, they have generated a picture of a dependent, feminine role, and have quickly become clichés as Sarosi has emphasized in a recent article.[2] The concept of the "mother surrogate" also has limited usefulness in describing the current role of the nurse.[3] It is a concept that has been overused and seems also to have contributed to a "housewife" kind of image of nurses.

Nurses in community mental health centers are functioning in much wider capacities than these. The above concepts of the nurse's role have done little to stimulate new theoretical knowledge, have not contributed toward nurses being viewed as intellectuals in the professional community or to their being fully utilized in the community mental health movement. Two recent studies indicate that nurses are not readily received as peers by other disciplines in the community mental health center.[4,5] As newcomers to the community mental health scene, nurses must undergo certain *rites de passage*, demonstrate their competence, and carve a place for themselves in the structure.

THE ORGANIZATIONAL STRUCTURE

The role of nurses cannot be described in simple terms; it is defined in part by the system in which they work, in part by the relationships they have with significant others, and in part by the nurse's individual personality and level of competence. In addition, the philosophy and structure of a system influence the degree of role expansion among all professionals, including nurses. Nurses have traditionally worked in rigid, hierarchical structures that are based on the medical model. The community mental health structure is different; it is not without its pecking order, but its philosophy tends to be more egalitarian, and its structure less rigid and hierarchical.

The organizational structure is nonetheless complex, as demonstrated by the diagram of the Mental Health Center of Denver General Hospital (see p. 8). As the diagram shows, nurses are involved at nearly every level and in every phase of our community mental health center. Furthermore, nurses participate in top and middle management positions as well as in hospital, day hospital, outpatient and emergency departments, consultation and education, and research elements. Additional elements of the fully comprehensive program are: specialized diagnostic and referral services; rehabilitation; precare and aftercare; and professional training and education. Again, nurses in our mental health center are involved both directly and indirectly in all these elements; and this involvement is probably unique in the country.

The relationship of the mental health center to the community and its needs is another important aspect which affects the role of the nurse. The community served by the Center is primarily an urban area: 60 percent of the population has an income of less than $6,000 per year; 50 percent of the population is composed of minority ethnic groups. The population of the Center's primary catchment area is about 200,000. However, all 530,000 citizens of Denver are eligible for service at Denver General Hospital, so the population actually served by the Division of Psychiatric Services is much larger than that of the Center's primary catchment area. The population of the primary catchment area is characterized by their low socioeconomic status, high rates of welfare recipiency, unemployment, police arrest and other indices of social dysfunction, and all types of mental illness.

Functionally, the Community Mental Health Center is operated with six decentralized generic outpatient teams and a centralized hospital and day hospital program.* Other specialized back-up services (such as psychiatric crisis services, psychological testing, diagnostic and referral service, research and education services) are also centralized in the hospital. Rehabilitation services

---

*"Generic" refers to the basic unit or the team which is located in the neighborhood catchment area.

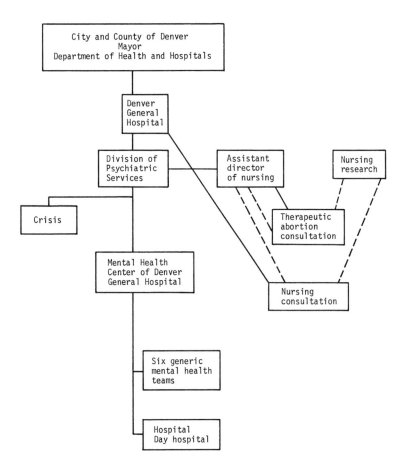

and services for therapeutic abortion applicants are delivered both centrally and by the outpatient team. A new comprehensive program for alcoholics and drug abusers will include centralized (detoxification center and intensive care units) and decentralized services given by personnel deployed to generic outpatient teams. While the organization of the Center is complex, it is operationally designed to provide readily available, high quality service to the residents of the primary catchment area and the city of Denver as well. Specialized services are centralized only when this seems to be the best way to provide high quality care.

The generic mental health team function as psychiatric general practitioners within a defined geographic catchment area. Each generic mental health team has roughly the same professional staff: a psychiatrist, a clinical psychologist, two psychiatric social workers, a psychiatric nurse, and a half-time rehabilitation counselor. Neighborhood aides and volunteers also work on the generic teams.

The philosophy of the center is that each generic team is responsible for seeing all patients, both adults and children, as soon as possible after their initial request for services. A powerful mandate guides our service delivery system: "Thou shalt have no waiting list." This mandate puts into operation our philosophical goal of providing readily available services.

The kinds of clinical and consultative programs that each team develops differ, depending on the needs of the community the team serves. For instance, one generic team serves a predominantly Mexican-American, poor working class or welfare population. In order to provide readily available service to this group, it was found that not only could no waiting list be entertained—there could be no appointments either. Therefore, this team has developed a drop-in clinic staffed by a neighborhood aide and a senior member of the professional staff.

A wide variety of treatment modalities are utilized at the Center. Traditional modalities include individual therapy, group therapy, and the therapeutic community. However, new modes are growing from each of the modalities. Family therapy, crisis therapy, reality therapy, behavior therapy and many specialized therapeutic groups are being expanded and used in programs that have been developed to meet the needs of large populations of deprived people.

The role of nurses in these various treatment modalities is limited only by their interests and capabilities. In other settings, the participation of nurses frequently is limited by the very fact that they are nurses. The concept of the nurse as the handmaiden to the doctor is only gradually disappearing. A former director of a community mental health center in Colorado, when questioned by a study group about how he planned to use nurses, very candidly stated that he had never thought of using them in an outpatient setting.[6] Having only observed nurses function on inpatient services, he felt that in an outpatient setting housewives could do the job. He did not see the nurse capable of functioning as an independent professional in any outpatient treatment modalities. Nurses in our Center, however, function in all settings with a great deal of role expansion resulting.

THE NURSE IN THE SYSTEM

Nurses' special functions in a community mental health center lie in their relationship to the patients, the team, and the community. Because of their "total patient" background and orientation, they remain the last of a vanishing breed, the generalist. Although nurses in the community mental health center have become specialized through graduate education or experience, their ability to relate to the patient as a total human being is prominent and distinct. We have seen nurses relate to patients in a less rigidly defined manner than do members of other disciplines. Furthermore, nurses seem to be more comfortable in implementing new, and eclectic methods of therapy. This flexibility is an absolute necessity for working with a socially deprived population which rarely responds to traditional methods of treatment.

Despite this "flexible, eclectic manner," four distinct roles of the nurse in community psychiatry, identified in a study at Denver General Community Mental Health Center in 1969, can be delineated: therapist, team member, liaison person for the patient and community agencies, and consultant.[7] Describing the role of the nurses in these terms is more explicit and professional than describing their role as "care, cure, coordination" or "mother surrogate." These roles are in the traditional areas of community mental health services—inpatient, emergency, and outpatient treatment. In less traditional areas such as team administration, working with therapeutic abortion general hospital nursing consultation, and nursing research, these four roles are also clear.

INPATIENT SERVICES. The role of the nurse on the inpatient service is primarily that of a therapist. In the therapeutic community milieu, nurses are active in a variety of group therapies which include psychodrama, small group therapy, community meetings, and recreational activities. In addition, the nurse is active in relating inpatient treatment to outpatient and other services in the center.

EMERGENCY SERVICES. The psychiatric emergency service is staffed primarily by nurses who carry the bulk of the treatment load. Nurses have assumed responsibility for assessment and preliminary diagnosis of psychiatric patients and their families. They make independent decisions with a minimum of consultation, conduct crisis therapy on an immediate and continuing basis, and make use of a wide variety of community resources in treating psychiatric patients. In this critical area where a high degree of clinical expertise and independent decision-making is required, the role of the nurse has become nearly indistinguishable from that of the psychiatrist.

OUTPATIENT SERVICES. As active members of treatment teams, the outpatient nurses are involved in a variety of therapeutic modalities. One nurse does a great deal of play therapy with children, and also conducts family therapy; this nurse's catchment area has many lower middle class families. Another nurse has established "hippie" groups, homosexual groups, and resocialization groups in boarding homes. On another team, servicing mobile, transient population, the nurse spends a great deal of time in the drop-in clinic where her function may vary from obtaining prescriptions for long-term patients to intervening with crisis therapy.

As nurses practice in community mental health centers, they quickly learn that the demand for service is greater than the supply of professionals. Utilization of numerous community agencies is vital in providing treatment for patients as well as in maintaining one's own sanity in a community mental health setting that forbids waiting lists. The most frequent contacts with the community include those with welfare personnel, visiting nurse services, juvenile authorities, the police, churches, other hospitals, schools, and neighborhood action committees. Nurse consultation to these agencies is used to promote therapeutic relationships between the caregiver and the client, increasing the caregiver's skill in caring for psychiatric patients, and encourage early case-finding.

TEAM ADMINISTRATION. Nurses in the outpatient setting are increasing in number throughout the country, but the nurse as an outpatient team leader is rare. The equalitarian goals of the therapeutic community notwithstanding, rank ascribed according to profession, not to education or to individual expertise, is a fact of life. The pecking order is found in community mental health centers as well as in chicken coops, and, more often than not, the nurse is lowest in the order.[8] All things can change, however, in even the medical model.

What happens when a nurse is appointed team leader? The earth "doth shake and tremble," but maintains its essential shape, and so does the nurse and the team, and the team leaders in other disciplines. In our setting, a nurse who was recently appointed team leader has assumed administrative and clinical responsibility while medical responsibility has remained with the psychiatrists. The nurse is responsible for assessing the community's needs and then tailoring clinical and consultative programs to meet those needs. Liaison work with other institutions and community agencies, assessment of the needs of the team, creation and maintenance of a cohesive, effective working group, as well as maintenance of her own clinical caseload are her responsiblities. She is also responsible for articulating the goals of the agency at the operational level.

THERAPEUTIC ABORTION PROGRAM. Another example of a program developed to meet a community need and an innovative role function of the nurse, is the therapeutic abortion program at Denver General Hospital. Implementation of a liberal abortion law in Colorado in 1967 created such problems as fragmentation of services, staff conflict, lack of psychiatric follow-up, and negative attitudes about abortion that affected patient care. A nurse has become the key person in this program, acting as liaison, consultant, and therapist, and has contributed toward making a therapeutic abortion truly therapeutic.

Consultation: Hospital Liaison Service

Too frequently we ignore problems in our own backyard to look at the problems next door. This is often true of community mental health centers located in general hospitals. A hospital experience is stressful and can be a destructive, regressive experience for a medical-surgical patient. Furthermore, many patients with psychiatric problems are hospitalized in general units. Both the "normal" and the psychiatric patient can act out under the stress of hospitalization and pose problems in management for the general hospital nursing staff. Our nursing consultation program was established to help nurses in the general hospital deal with these problems more effectively.

In order to decrease the barrier that often exists between general hospital and psychiatric nursing staff the members of the consultation group have made themselves available on a 24-hour, seven-day-a-week basis. Methods used by the nurse consultants have varied from a direct crisis intervention with a patient to formal group consultation with the nursing staff on a one-time or continuing basis.

To cite an example, a brief crisis consultation occurred when a staff nurse called at 1:00 A.M. A patient's mood had changed suddenly from manic excitement to depressed withdrawal and the nurse wanted to discuss what might be the most effective approach to the patient. Longer term consultation has been provided in such instances as the outpatient obstetrical nurses asking for help in dealing with "hippies." Several weeks of group discussion with a member of the "hip community" as a resource person, promoted greater understanding of and effectiveness in dealing with the "hippie."

The consultation service has helped the general hospital nursing staff achieve a better understanding of patients' problem behavior and greater skill in dealing with many kinds of "problem patients." Since no other member of the psychiatric team can fully understand the difficulties and complexities of the nurse's work on a general hospital unit, the consultation has been provided most effectively by a psychiatric nurse.

Research

Too frequently nursing research has been left to other disciplines, and often the results have had little applicable value to the practicing nurse. Research by any discipline in a community mental health setting must be useful to both the community and those who serve it. Discussing research and developing new studies were our primary goals in establishing a psychiatric nursing research conference group. Its purpose was twofold: (1) to stimulate writing and research by individual nurses; and (2) to plan, initiate, and complete projects as a group. The nursing consultation program discussed above is such a group endeavor.

The nurse in research has expanded her role from one of assistant to that of an independent primary investigator. At present she receives consultation from peers as well as from experts in research. She collaborates with others from the Division of Psychiatric Services in carrying out projects such as investigating the effect of a stillbirth, or neonatal death during the last trimester of pregnancy. Designing and implementing nursing studies, for example, analyzing the role of the nurse in our community mental health center and evaluating the effectiveness of the nursing consultation program illustrate the developing role of the nurse in research.

SUMMARY

Nurses have been agents of change in the Mental Health Center of Denver General Hospital, both for their professional group and for the total system. With their generalist orientation and their practical flexibility, nurses have much to contribute to community mental health practice. They can be parental surrogates but in the community mental health center context, this description is limited—as a label and as a guide for nursing practice. Nurses do "care," they do "cure," and they do "coordinate." But they do so in the more sophisticated context of therapist, team leader, liaison, and consultant.

REFERENCES

1. American Nurses Association: A Position Paper. New York, The Association, 1965, p. 5.
2. Sarosi, G.M. A critical theory: the nurse as a fully human person. Nursing Forum, 7:349, 1968.
3. Peplau, H.E. Interpersonal Relations in Nursing, A Conceptual Frame of Reference for Psychodynamic Nursing. New York, G.P. Putnam's Sons, 1952, Chap. 3.
4. Glittenberg, J. The role of the nurse in the outpatient psychiatric clinic. Amer. J. Orthopsychiat., 33:713, July, 1963.
5. Stokes, G.A., Williams, F.S., Davidites, R.M., Bulbulyan, A., and Ullman, M. The Roles of Psychiatric Nurses in Community Mental Health Practice: A Giant Step. Maimonides Medical Center——Community Mental Health Center , 1969.
6. De Young, C., Tower, M., et al. The Nurse's Role in Community Mental Health Centers Out of Uniform and into Trouble. St. Louis, The C.V. Mosby Co., 1971.
7. Zahourek, R. Analysis of the Role of the Nurse in a Community Mental Health Center. unpublished study, Denver General Hospital, Division of Psychiatric Services, 1969.
8. De Young and Tower, op. cit.

BIBLIOGRAPHY

ANA, Psychiatric-Mental Health Nursing Division. Statement On Psychiatric Nursing: Developmental Statement, New York, American Nurses Association, 1967.
Gregg, D.E. The therapeutic roles of the nurse. Perspect. Psychiat. Care, 1:18, 1963.
King, S.H. Perceptions of Illness and Medical Practice. New York, Russell Sage Foundation, 1962, p. 241.
Leininger, M.M. Community psychiatric nursing: trends, issues and problems. Perspect. Psychiat. Care, 7:10, 1969.

Mereness, D. The potential significant role of the nurse in community mental
    health services. Perspect. Psychiat. Care, 3:34, 1963.
Sheldon, A. and Hope, P.K. The developing role of the nurse in a community
    mental health program. Perspect. Psychiat. Care, 5:272, 1967.
White, O.H., Bloch, D.W., Glittenberg, J., Nehrer, J.G., and Smith, K.M. Nursing
    in Community Mental Health Services. NIMH Pilot Project, University of
    Colorado, 1967.

DISCUSSION*

Question:

You described the individual team's power in terms of planning and administering services. You also mentioned a central executive administration. How did nursing get involved in the overall policy-making level?

Miss Tower:

We used power and pushed to get the nurse in at the central administrative level. As a group we met and formulated the rationale for nursing input at the decision-making level. So often, I think nurses just go along in the service roles, and wonder about the lack of accomplishment. When we started getting involved at the executive level, we realized that we needed that additional power to support and help bring about changes in nursing practice at the team level. Nurses combined their ingenuity and practicality in negotiating for space in the community. The community mental health teams operate in the local catchment area, maintaining offices in churches, reconverted office buildings, and in neighborhood health centers. We have two large and one small neighborhood health centers, each housing a mental health team. One of the teams is still in the hospital. If we can get the bureaucracy moving, that team will be in the community too. The psychiatric emergency team is in the hospital emergency room, covering all six areas.

Question:

What provision have you for communication between the nurses and the other mental health staff on the six teams that are located in the community?

Miss Tower:

This hasn't been too much of a problem. There are weekly staff meetings in each section; that is, each team, inpatient, outpatient, and psychiatric emergency room service has its own staff meetings. In addition, we have a total staff meeting once a week. I, personally, meet with the nurses in the outpatient and other service modalities, and join in staff meetings and meetings out in the

*Note—Miss Tower presented and discussed this paper. Her co-author Mrs. Zahourek partici-
pated in another group.

community in order to keep in touch. Nursing staff in each area meet once a month. These meetings keep communication open. However, as agency staff reaches upwards of 300, communication becomes more difficult.

Comment:

You indicated that your satellite clinics were staffed with professional members. We've started self-help clinics in two communities, using people in the community who have the interest, know-how, and ability. We utilize our new careerists in these self-help centers and the professionals serve as consultants. We have extended our roles through the paraprofessional, which has enabled us to supply relevant services. This endeavor has been professionally rewarding as found power from below, which made it possible to counterbalance the power from above. We were able to change policies and reorder priorities to coincide with what the client was experiencing.

Question:

You were talking about consultation to the staff in the general hospital and other agencies. Would you tell us more about that?

Miss Tower:

The nurses in the inpatient setting are more involved in consultation to other nurses in the hospital and are minimally involved in consultation with other community groups. The nurses in the outpatient settings are more involved in consultation with other groups within the agency and within the community, both on an informal and formal basis. The rest of us in administration, research, and the therapeutic abortion program are involved in both; the therapeutic abortion program is a specialized consultative process which involves primarily direct services to the client and limited consultation to the agency personnel. There is a specialized program developing now for school-age children. The nurse is one of the primary members of that team and is planning to work with teachers, and parents of disturbed children.

Comment:

I was interested to hear you say that community mental health nurses are concerned and involved in research. In my agency we have tripartite responsibility for teaching, research, and clinical practice. One of the complaints is that, considering the pressures on the nurses arising from their involvement in the community, research has received minimal attention. It's very encouraging to have heard your report.

Miss Tower:

What made the difference in our program was having one nurse with primary responsibility in the area of research. She was able to coordinate the research project and do the rough draft writing. When we asked who would be interested in participating in research, nurses from all settings volunteered. The group consists of about 10 or 15 nurses involved in this project on a strictly voluntary basis. This project would not have been possible without a nurse researcher.

Question:

Do the nursing practitioners have faculty appoints in the university?

Miss Tower:

No, because it's politically complicated. The general hospital split with the medical school about six years ago. We at the general hospital are community oriented and the psychiatric department of the medical school is analytically oriented. It raises an interesting point between educators and clinicians about status. I was determined, when I went to the general hospital from a teaching position at the university, that I was not going to be viewed as a second-class citizen since there were excellently prepared clinical practitioners at the general hospital. We plan and provide workshops. We're involved in the university now but do not have faculty appointments.

I just wanted to say one thing about where we are in terms of nursing in our center. We've made use of a lot of things, mainly our competence. We weren't always where we are today, as far as nursing goes. Four years ago the only nurse to be found was in the inpatient unit. We started out with two graduate students on two outpatient teams who demonstrated that they were capable of working in a variety of settings and with various treatment modalities. Now, nurses are involved in the system because they could do the job that needed to be done, they've become a very strong department, and are well-respected professionals within the system. The nurses are considered one of the strongest professional groups in the community mental health center because they've demonstrated their ability to expand their role. It can be done—it takes money and a director who's interested in new programs and really moves. However, the most important thing is that the nurses can do it.

Comment:

You are suggesting that competency brings power. Competency is necessary but it is not enough; you have to look to someone else for the money and the sanction to work and you have to know how to maneuver to get that.

Comment:

We've been talking about some unique qualities of nursing. We've used the term "patient," we've used "client" occasionally, and whenever we've talked about groups, they have been labeled as "ill." In lieu of this discussion, I was hoping we would evolve a role of the nurse as a caretaker who has access to "well populations." While much of what nurses are doing has had many innovative qualities to it, it seems as though we're still pathology-oriented. Even the consultation in schools sounded like it was still dealing with pathology.

Comment:

To be frank, we are still in a hassle regarding the philosophy in our program. Is our role that of a community psychiatry center, service-oriented, caring for the psychiatric patient? Or is it that of a community mental health center oriented to preventive care, that is, social action. Or is that someone else's job? Should our primary goal be to take care of people or to deal with the social environment? There is some split about this and there's going to be a lot more discussion before it is resolved. One rationale is that in our society we're always going to have psychiatric patients and someone needs to take care of them and "we can't do everything," that is, take care of them and prevent the problems at the same time. Where is our main focus going to be?

Comment:

It's not an "either—or," it's a "both." I think there should be a part of the center that would relate to the illness aspect, and another part to deal with prevention.

Comment:

I don't really see a polarization between the two goals. I see them on a continuum, in terms of primary, secondary, and tertiary prevention. Community mental health centers are supposed to be doing all three types of prevention ranging from health and health-maintenance to illness.

Comment:

I'd like to comment on that because I think that mental health centers can and ought to do both, but there *is* a problem with polarization. The assumption is that if we do one, then automatically, that eliminates the other. At our agency, we have the same split. We have people who give lip service to the notion that we should be involved in the community, but when it comes to really getting down to work, the people who are really out there are the nurses. And we carry a few of the psychiatrists with us.

Comment:

We talked about the process of consultation and the phases the consultee has to go through to understand how to use the therapeutic relationship. I think nurses and maybe all of the mental health workers are in the process of moving away from something that is concrete and comfortable—therapy, with one, two, or more patients—to something that's much more abstract, dealing with identifying the community as the client-at-large, in terms of consultation; and social change, that is, change from within the agency; and social action, that is, change from the community. I'm not just speaking about nursing because nursing is in the community—I'm talking about the institution within which nursing is working. We hear statements like, "We realize that there are things out there which interfere with the kinds of things we are trying to do for patients in here but we *must* limit ourselves to those things that we know how to do and we don't know anything about that out there." I say, as an institution, you plan a program and you find people who do know.

Question:
I could conceive of mental health centers having a division, just as there are other divisions, called the "political-legal division." It would deal with political and legal issues as a division of community mental health because in many aspects of our work there is a need for legal consultation. To give you an example, we have a drug dependency program and sometimes we have people on the units who are being detoxified, and we have legal authorities coming in to serve papers. We also have indigenous workers and legal problems occur in relation to them. What legal rights do employees and clients have? We need clarification in dealing with these problems.

Comment:
These kinds of experiences concern us. We don't necessarily know the answers; however, we need to have legal counsel. We have a responsibility to help people, to identify their needs, to identify alternative approaches to meeting them, to appraise them of the pros and cons of one alternative over the other. For example, this could conceivably be a group of welfare mothers who are going to march on City Hall and we need to have somebody to help them plan the best strategy to get their needs met. Whether we go with them, whether they go to jail, whether we go to jail with them; all these questions occur and we don't have the proper consultants. Ultimately, we will know how to help groups organize and anticipate some of the consequences of their action. We will identify the limits of staff's participation and state it clearly so that client groups will not have unrealistic expectations from us.

Comment:
In our agency we have a forensic psychiatry team that deals with these problems.

Comment:
We ought to have this service in the general hospitals as well but certainly it is needed in the community mental health centers.

Comment:

We have a program such as you mentioned, but there are still problems with it. The clinical and nonclinical services are at odds with each other. The nonclinical group has developed community organization skills and brought people on the staff to give that kind of service. However, the clinical services are not referring clients to them for help. We all share information with each other and become a huge information-sharing group. The nurse needs to gain this knowledge. My question is, "How much can I absorb?"

Comment:

Another problem is that everybody doesn't have to do everything or be expert in everything—it is the total picture of the insititution which is the most important. The new careers program is the first place that we've instituted knowledge of social systems in a concrete way. One of the things that perhaps the groups in institutions need to look at is the social systems as they relate to mental health—to understand the dynamics of the systems; and to understand social systems theory. It's not just social action versus treatment, and psychiatry ought not be involved in all kinds of social action. We need to learn what are some of the areas of social systems that have a tremendous impact on health of the individuals in the community. Whether one works with systems within or outside the institution, one must be aware of the political realities and of the legislative processes that are available in order to achieve goals. You might find, unless you know how to make constructive use of those processes, that funds dry up.

The Role of the Community Mental Health Nurse in a Rural Setting

JUSTINA D. NEUFELD, R.N., B.S.

This paper is based on my experience with the Mid-Kansas Rural Aftercare Demonstration at Prairie View Mental Health Center, Newton, Kansas. The project, sponsored by the National Institute of Mental Health (Grant Number 5-R01 MH 14977), began in 1964 and terminated in 1969. Since that time I have been a member of the Prairie View tri-county clinical team.

The setting for the aftercare demonstration was a tri-county area in central Kansas (Harvey, McPherson and Marion Counties) with a combined population of 65,000. The area is semirural; most of its people live in small towns. However, about 20 percent of our patients are quite isolated. A patient living in a rural area does experience his world differently from a patient, for example, living in New York City. It seems to me that a psychotic person is more visible in a rural area. If Mrs. C goes to the grocery store in the county seat and acts inappropriately it may be only a matter of hours before the word is spread in the community that she is "unbalanced." Often the center may be contacted for advice on what to do about Mrs. C, or the police or county sheriff may be contacted and Mrs. C brought to the community mental health center.

Mrs. C's world on the farm is different from a large, urban world because there are days and days when she sees no one except her husband. Her world revolves around him. As Mrs. C sits by her window looking out on mile after mile of prairie, she may begin to feel her isolation from humanity. For the visiting nurse, the miles of driving before meeting another car or passing another farm, can be very lonely but also very useful. It gives her time for reflection and preparation prior to the next visit.

Prairie View is a private nonprofit center which serves the tri-county catchment area on a contract basis.[1] On a private basis the center serves a much larger area. The total staff of about 110 includes ten psychiatric nurses, four psychiatrists, four psychologists, and eight psychiatric social workers.

Prairie View offers all the elements of a comprehensive community mental health service. Its program operates on the premise that mental health and mental illness are the responsibility of the total community and not the special property of any vested interest or group. Staff members are encouraged to utilize their potentials as fully as possible. Although traditional mental health specialist roles are recognized, staff members are encouraged to develop to the level of their capability, regardless of the discipline they represent.

Since the project terminated, our goal for the aftercare project and for community services has been to provide low-cost services while emphasizing group approaches and referrals to existing agencies. We have sought to accomplish these goals within a minimum amount of professional mental health worker time and have attempted to structure a program which would be adaptable in other rural areas and that eventually could be carried by agencies existing in a given geographical location. We have attempted to stimulate community concern for mental health problems, and encourage individuals and groups to assume greater responsibility for persons who manifest symptoms of behavioral disorder.

At the conclusion of the project last June, the aftercare function was absorbed by a tri-county clinical team consisting of a psychiatrist, social worker, community mental health nurse, part-time community aide, and some volunteers. Aftercare activities include monthly group meetings for patients and their families, a medication clinic, and a home visiting program. These activities are supplemented by individual and group psychotherapy. We have discovered a greater demand for nursing services in our aftercare program that we had originally anticipated.

EVOLVING ROLE

One finds frequent mention of the unidentified role of the nurse on a community mental health team in the literature. Mereness writes that many a nurse finds herself in an uncertain situation when she accepts a position on a psychiatric team.[2] The usual hope is that the role of the nurse can be defined as the staff work together in meeting patient needs. Patient needs do help to define roles, but when roles are allowed to emerge in such a way, usually one of three roles is assigned to the nurse—that of receptionist, of visiting in the home and focusing on the physical problems, or of extending the role of some other member of the team. In retrospect, I can say that all of these roles were, at one time or another, assigned to me. I was, however, given the freedom to add to or reject aspects of the evolving role, and at times this lead to a great deal of anxiety for me. It seemed that my struggle with role identification for the community mental health nurse was intensified by the fact that the more traditional nursing role also is changing.

Although my previous experience included working in a provincial mental hospital, a tuberculosis sanitarium, a general hospital admission ward, and, for five years, the Prairie View inpatient psychiatric service, I was not prepared for what I was to learn as a community mental health nurse. Much of the time I worked relatively independently, and my role began to overlap extensively with the roles of other center staff members. I found myself working with community agencies, who had similar goals for a given patient, and who were going about achieving these goals in very different ways. I learned by doing.

In 1964 I prepared the following role description of the aftercare nurse:

1. To provide medication, supervision, and nursing care, carrying out recommendations made by physician or psychiatrist.
2. To assist with various kinds of physical care, providing instructions in such areas as sanitation, hygiene, housekeeping, diet, and caring for both children and the aged.
3. To ease apprehensions and correct superstitions and other erroneous concepts held by patients and their families relating to mental illness.
4. To assist in dealing with housing problems which ranged from talks with landlords and neighbors to assistance to patients and their families in finding new living quarters or new living arrangements such as foster homes or boarding homes.
5. To help provide, through community resources, legal aid for patients requiring such help.
6. To help patients with employment problems.
7. To help patients adjust to their new environment by interpreting resources available in the community and assisting patients in joining appropriate recreational, church, and social groups.
8. To encourage self-reliance, and to give support by listening.
9. To act as a liaison among the mental health team members.

During the course of the project I found myself functioning in all of these ways. As a project nurse, I worked closely with the co-director during the minimal contact and medication clinics, and devoted a major portion of my time to home visits. My other duties included keeping systematic records of patient contacts and acting as a liaison between team members and community agencies. It soon became clear that the role of the community mental health center nurse is, and of necessity must be, an evolving one. It emerges as a result of center goals, team goals, and the continuous process of interaction among the team members. As the team applies itself to getting the job done, meeting specific needs is matched to the time and ability of team members. It is through this process that the nurse's role gradually emerges.

Establishing and Maintaining Contact

RECEIVING REFERRALS. The categories of persons referred to the nurse for contact in home, office, or medication clinic were the following: (1) persons who were felt to have special needs or who may have been treated in any of the other treatment center modalities; (2) persons who would not or could not come to the clinic, possibly because of transportation problems, health, or anxiety; (3) persons needing close drug supervision; (4) persons being maintained in the community by supportive care; (5) persons who had linkage with other community resources; (6) persons unresponsive to more formal therapeutic encounters who were unable to introspect or communicate effectively orally; (7) persons whose families were involved in their illnesses but were not receptive to treatment at the clinic.

Generally, referrals to the nurse were made on an informal basis. Some patients were introduced to the nurse while still in the hospital, others were met at the clinic on referral from Topeka (Kansas) State Hospital. As the nurse's role became better known, referrals from county social welfare workers, nursing home administrators, and public health nurses increased. A few referrals came from physicians in the community after the nurse had developed a relationship with them. Several patients referred themselves after hearing about the service. On several occasions patients told the nurse about other discharged patients. These leads were followed by inquiries to the Topeka State Hospital team.

ESTABLISHING CONTACT. As any visiting nurse knows, there are certain implications in the home visitation concept. Meeting the person on home territory implies dealing with the total milieu, not just one person in the home. When she enters a home the nurse moves into private territory, sometimes without invitation, and at times her presence may barely be tolerated. Entering the home is entering the patient's world. As one Topeka State Hospital team member put it in discussing discharge plans for a person with a history of repeated admissions and particularly difficult problems, "But this time it will be different; I can just see that nurse walking behind him as he is plowing the field, trying to get him to take his medication." The nurse never had the occasion to walk behind the plow with a cup of pills but the fantasy is not far from reality.

At times it was impossible to reach the patient directly and numerous indirect routes had to be taken before a relationship could be established. Follow-up contacts have taken me to the barn where a patient's husband was working, to parsonages to talk with pastors, and to other resource persons such as lawyers, guardians, landlords, public health nurses, employers, and social welfare workers. All the nurse takes into these situations is herself and her ability to relate to the patient *in his environment* with the goal of helping him to develop more effective patterns of living.

Not every nurse will be able to relate comfortably to the wide range of professionals and nonprofessionals who are involved with the patient's environment in the community. However, it is essential that one member of the team is able to extend himself in such a way that he may actually act in behalf of, or speak for, the patient whose language and behavior repertoire is limited. Why not the nurse who, because of her traditional standing, has enjoyed more direct access to the community?

PURSUIT TACTICS. There is more to effective aftercare than merely keeping the former state hospital patient in the community. Freeman and Simmons define the successfully rehabilitated person as "the one who is able to live in a nonmedical setting at a level of occupational and social performance comparable with that of other adults in the community."[3]

Considering the fact that most patients already have been exposed to years of treatment, the above goal may seem too lofty. Not only may they manifest chronic mental health problems, but often they also represent the lowest socioeconomic stratum in the population. They may come from disorganized or multiproblem families—families who are known to various agencies in their community. They do not share middle-class values, symbols, and modes of communication. Since typically they are acquainted less well with formal ways of doing things than are middle-class persons, less can be left to chance in communicating with them.

When those we are serving lose contact with us either through design or by default, we turn to "pursuit tactics." The cliché that is often used, "they will find us when they need us," usually does not hold true for the poorly integrated person. Although he probably will come back to a given agency after a gross disturbance or after a relapse has occurred, the fact is that he often does not find help when he needs it.

Pursuit tactics have been used effectively in public health to deal with epidemics, cancer, and tuberculosis. But those of us in the mental health field seem slow to learn from the prevention experiences of general medicine. When the mentally ill person is returned to the community, he is referred frequently to a helping agency; but, for various reasons, meaningful contact may never be established. Typically an aggressive effort is not made to track down the previously hospitalized person. Pursuit may be seen as an important mental health center task. With her training and experience in working directly with people, the nurse appears to be specially qualified to contribute in this area. (An exemplary case study appears in Appendix A.)

MAINTAINING MOTIVATION. After the initial enthusiasm associated with a new project has worn off, the visiting nurse faces the grim reality that the majority of persons with whom she works are low-keyed, often unexciting, even unpleasant, and chronically ill persons who will not achieve any dramatic changes. And—it is hard work to carry the responsibility for maintaining contact with such clients.

In my case, motivation was maintained by: (1) support from the mental health center team; (2) attending workshops and meetings with people from various other disciplines; (3) expanding my mental health service skills—working with a married couples' group of less chronically ill persons; and (4) working experiences with volunteers and nursing students. Students are eager idealists. They often are shocked by the realities, but they seem to have an optimistic resiliency. Volunteers bring in new and refreshing ideas, and sometimes approach problems quite differently than do paid mental health center staff members.

Community Involvement

COMMUNITY RESOURCE COUNCIL. Early during the aftercare venture, it became apparent that some of the patients in the program were known to numerous other community helping agencies. Representatives from the various agencies began to meet to help one another to deal with difficult cases. Several case conferences were held and members felt they were beneficial to both client and agencies. When we agreed to hold regular interagency meetings, the Community Resource Council was born.

The Council evolved out of the aftercare program. However, it required a tremendous amount of energy to keep the various agencies involved on a continuing basis, especially when a given agency felt no particular crisis that directly called for interagency communication. It became my responsibility to maintain contact with the various agencies for the purpose of keeping the council alive and productive. In retrospect, the effort was worthwhile; the Resource Council has functioned effectively. My ongoing relationship with representatives from the social welfare departments, public health departments, school counseling programs, the ministerial alliance, employment agencies, probate courts, the sheriff's offices, and other helping agencies continues to be a real asset.

As a result of joint planning, new services have emerged. Some of them are particularly important for former patients; others are for the benefit of the community in general. An experiment with a group for single parents was conducted; the home extension office established a program of instruction in basic homemaking for a group of women who are in the poor or "nonclubbing" class; families of former state hospital patients as well as others in the community have made use of the program. (See case study in Appendix B.)

SUMMARY

As a result of our experience with the aftercare demonstration and the subsequent broader community services program, we have learned several things. First, it is clear that the role of the community nurse in a mental health center is an evolving one. What began as a nursing role in an experimental aftercare project has resulted in an ongoing role with outpatients for a community mental health nurse in a comprehensive mental health center setting. Second, it has become obvious that those who most need help often cannot reach out to find it. Pursuit needs to be a part of the ongoing program of the comprehensive mental health center, and the nurse is specially qualified to play a central role in this task. Third, we learned something about the way in which nurses can become involved with a community in its task of meeting mental health needs. We have attempted to share these learnings in a short-term, intensive program for community nurses (See Appendix C). My experience with this expanding nursing role has been a step-by-step process of increasing personal involvement in the task of strengthening and maintaining community mental health resources.

APPENDIX A

The following case illustrates three particular problem areas: (1) mental health center staff members tend to be reluctant to pursue patients aggressively in the community; however, in many situations, pursuit tactics are essential to preventive treatment and to continuity of care; (2) the team had obvious difficulty in deciding which member of the interdisciplinary team should pursue the case; assignments had to be made in the light of patient needs, professional skills, personal talents, and time available; and (3) it is very difficult to maintain contact with a patient when there are constant barriers raised by the patient or his family. It is hard to give when not directly requested to give.

Mrs. C called the community mental health center identifying herself as having been in Topeka State Hospital at one time and asking if she could talk to someone. She talked briefly with the aftercare team social worker and was given a clinic appointment the following day. However the next day she called the receptionist to cancel the appointment stating she didn't need to come in. At the social worker's request the nurse followed up the cancellation with a phone call asking if she might visit in the home. Mrs. C seemed to have difficulty making a decision but finally said, "I'll ask my husband when he comes home from work." The phone conversation revealed that Mrs. C was hallucinating regularly. She stated she was feeling like she had before entering the hospital. She had had three previous state hospital admissions, two of which had been longer than two years. She stated that she always felt strange when she was not taking her pills. The following day the nurse called again to inquire if she might make a home visit. Mrs. C replied that her husband would allow the nurse to visit "one time."

When the nurse visited, Mrs. C's appearance was untidy and her house was in disarray. She displayed some anxiety, touching her legs and arms randomly, probably in an attempt to control her anxiety. She communicated to the nurse that she was afraid of her husband so she isolated herself. In her isolation she found a great deal of satisfaction in listening to the "voices" that would reassure her that they loved her. Before leaving, the nurse encouraged Mrs. C to take her pills as prescribed and said she would contact Mr. C to obtain his consent to visit again.

The following day the nurse placed a person-to-person call to Mr. C at his place of employment and also called his home. No contact was made with him that day or after repeated attempts during the following week. In the meantime, the aftercare team had learned that the couple's adolescent son had been hospitalized at Prairie View several years earlier. At that time there had been difficulty in involving the parents and the account had never been paid. In short, there had been considerable frustration with the family before the son was eventually transferred to Topeka State Hospital. In discussing this with the team they were initially reluctant to become involved with this family again. The question was raised whether we shouldn't inform Topeka State Hospital about Mrs. C's relapse and since she was on convalescent leave, return her to the hospital. But the team felt that this was avoiding the real issues.

But—how were we to work with the family if there was no way of reaching the husband? Who of the team members should pursue this aspect? The team agreed that the nurse should continue her attempts to get in touch with the family. They felt that the nurse might not threaten this man who already felt his inadequacies so keenly. Initially, when Mr. C was eventually contacted by phone, he was negative. He kept saying, "Expense is one thing I don't need and I don't see that she needs help. She always has my supper ready when I come home and that's all I ask." However, he reluctantly agreed to let the nurse visit again.

Mrs. C started taking her medications and in a month she was able to come to the monthly group and medication clinic at the center. She continued to hallucinate intermittently but began to show interest in her surroundings and in other people. Mr. C and the son avoided the nurse. The daughter lived quite a distance from home and never was available. When the nurse purposely arranged a visit on a Saturday so the husband could be present, he refused to come in from the pig barn. The patient was fearful about the nurse going to the barn saying "He has such a temper I don't know what he'll do to you."

Mrs. C then began looking for a job saying, "If I could earn $5 a month I wouldn't have to beg him for money." After three years, Mrs. C still is receiving aftercare. For the last year she has attended only the monthly group and medication clinic, and the visiting nurse has visited as necessary. A volunteer from the clinic also visits her once a month. However, she has had numerous crises: her only daughter was married; her infant grandson died; her adolescent son lost several jobs; and after the son and his wife moved out of the house the son had to declare bankruptcy. None of these crises required the patient's rehospitalization at Topeka State Hospital. Mr. C eventually agreed to let his wife work and she obtained a dishwashing job which she kept for about one year.

Mrs. C has gained little or no insight into the root of her problems; she does not understand how she contributes to her difficulty with her husband, nor is she aware of how she brings isolation on from the community herself. However, by working on concrete things such as organizing the household, planning the day, shopping, and using community resources, Mrs. C has regained the relatively stable adjustment which had been essential to this family's functioning in the past. She sees the clinic contact as the highlight of the month. Her husband no longer objects to her involvement with the community mental health center since she has been "her old self again," even earning her own money to pay the monthly $5 fee. By staying in the community, of course, she has saved the taxpayer a great deal of money. The nonmonetary values are more difficult to evaluate—but they are there.

APPENDIX B

The following case illustrates the intense struggle sometimes required by an attempt to involve the community—a struggle nonetheless necessary if the patient is to live as a responsible citizen once again.

Mrs. E, a 46-year-old woman from a small rural town, was referred for aftercare services after repeated hospitalizations for psychiatric illness. Her diagnosis was "mild mental deficiency with schizophrenic reaction, chronic paranoid type." Mrs. E's first hospitalization took place during the ninth year of her marriage three weeks after the first child was born. Each of her several hospitalizations came when her symptoms took the form of excessive concern with "the communists taking over."

During Mrs. E's seventh admission, Mr. E did not visit or write to her for one year. Only after Mrs. E wrote repeatedly did he finally answer. She was doing well and the social worker encouraged her husband to consider taking her home on a trial visit, which he did. After the trial visit her husband conveyed the impression that it was o.k. if she were discharged but if she didn't come home that was o.k. also. He would make the best of either situation. He seemed quite comfortable that his wife had a home in the hospital, and he had made something of a life for himself and his daughter; in other words, he was satisfied without his wife. When he did not respond to any further overtures from the social worker to plan for his wife's discharge, the state hospital personnel, the local social welfare worker, and the Prairie View aftercare team met to discuss the case. They agreed that because of Mr. E's extreme passiveness the only way to proceed was to notify him that he must come for his wife on a certain date or she would be brought to his home. If no one was there to meet her, she would be taken to the local welfare office.

Under this kind of pressure Mr. E went to the state hospital at the designated time and brought his wife home. Prior to discharge, the state hospital social worker had talked with Mrs. E about the Prairie View visiting nurse coming to see her, and she accepted the idea readily. When the nurse made her first visit, Mrs. E was standing at the window waiting. She spent the given time talking about how she felt after having been gone for almost two years.

During the next three years, attempts were made to mobilize resources to assist Mrs. E to remain in the community. The first person the nurse approached was the pastor of Mrs. E's church. His response to the nurse's request to help Mr. E to provide transportation to the medication clinic seemed to express the feeling of Mrs. E's husband and the total community: "Frankly speaking, I don't think anybody wants her back. She is not an easy person to love; she is odd. We are always relieved when she goes back to the hospital. She is not very bright you know."

Eventually, Mrs. E was able to attend the monthly clinic. The social welfare worker provided transportation a number of times, and the nurse made home visits weekly. Mrs. E improved in spite of the fact that the community expected her to fail. She has made considerable progress in the past four years, demonstrating that she can keep house, raise a garden, and do a great amount of vegetable canning. Often she has given produce to the neighbors. She has begun to make herself more attractive and has cared for her daughter's physical needs.

With support from the visiting nurse, Mrs. E has been able to function in spite of the rejection by her husband and the community. Gradually, in the past year, the community has become noticeably involved with Mrs. E and with others who are in need of some form of intervention.

APPENDIX C

COMMUNITY NURSING COURSE

A short-term intensive program for community nurses was an outgrowth of our experience in the first three years of the Prairie View aftercare project. A course entitled "Mental Health Principles in Community Nursing" was developed with the help of a grant from the Community Mental Health Section of the

Kansas State Board of Institutional Management. We had expected community nurses (as well as members of other helping agencies) to become involved quite naturally in the mental health aspects of the aftercare program as a result of increased communication about common concerns. They were invited to participate in monthly Resource Council meetings and in specific nurse-related responsibilities such as making home visits and helping with the monthly clinic. But we soon became aware of the high turnover rate of community nurses and of the fact that none of the nurses had had public health training. A few had had no psychiatric nursing experience at all.

Nurses' responses indicated a need for the course. These included: failing to attend Resource Council meetings when their specified areas of concern were discussed; making only one or two "investigative" home visits; not attempting to involve community resources; and perceiving the social and recreational hour as "silly." These reactions revealed a need to clarify expectations and mobilize a means of support which might help the nurses become vitally involved. The program that emerged was an attempt on our part to help the public health nurse develop her skills as a community mental health resource. An added impetus to offer the course for nurses came from my participation at the Boston Work Conference on Short Term Clinical Training of Nurses for Community Mental Health Centers in 1967.

When the Prairie View staff first began planning for community nurses, we assumed we could outline a training program that would be accepted readily by the recipients. However, in a meeting with area nurses, supervisors, the state director of public health nursing and the regional mental health nursing consultant, the necessity of making this a collaborative process at every level became clear. There was also a specific request that only nurses be involved in the program planning sessions. We proceeded in this way, using Prairie View staff from other disciplines on a consultative basis.

The enthusiasm of the students was evident during the first week of the program. It became a stimulating time for all who participated. The monthly half-day followup sessions were well attended also. These sessions dealt with a number of vital issues such as maintaining a patient at a minimum functioning level, and confrontation in the home situation. The nurse's role in the community was a critical issue for some. Case reports were presented for discussion. Programmed materials from the Human Development Institute in Atlanta dealing with human relations in nursing were utilized.[4] In general the experience demonstrated that the nurse can make an impact on the community by becoming involved with clients in a new way.

REFERENCES

1. Glasscote, R., Sanders, D., Forstenzer, H.M., and Foley, A.R. The Community Mental Health Center: An Analysis of Existing Models,

Washington, D.C., American Psychiatric Association, 1964, pp. 121-132.
2. Mereness, D. The potential significant role of the nurse in community mental health services. Perspect. Psychiat. Care, 1 (3):34, 1963.
3. Freeman, H.E., and Simmons, O.G. The Mental Patient Comes Home, New York, John Wiley & Sons, Inc., 1963.
4. Human Relations in Nursing Program, Revised Preliminary Edition, Atlanta, Human Development Institute, Inc., 1968.

DISCUSSION

Question:
What are the requirements for a successful aftercare program?

Miss Neufeld:
We have learned several things. One of the important ones was that personal contact with the state hospital personnel on a continuing basis facilitates mutual respect and trust which is necessary to the concept of continuity of care.

Other learnings included the need for an immediate intake procedure to 'hook' the patient to the aftercare program. This procedure includes establishing an initial relationship between the patient and the treatment team as well as the formulation of treatment plans with the patient and family members. Therapeutic alliance between the aftercare team and the patient and his family begins at this point.

The person who is beginning to arouse concern in community mental health practice is the person who cannot make his own way or doesn't have a protective 'living base' in which to stay. This has led us to believe that learning the social role function is a most important aspect of treatment. Related to this is the establishment of a kind of 'ecological niche' for the patient, and here we are referring to the physically and emotionally sheltered corner of the world where the person may live, have contact with other people, and fulfill as complex a role as he is capable of fulfilling.

Periodic contact with a person, or persons, in whom the patient has had trust over an indefinite period of time is important. Such contacts range from once a week to as little as ten minutes a month—but they serve to help the patient maintain himself in the community. People other than those trained in professional mental health work can be of help in giving support. We have had experience mostly with volunteer workers in these supportive roles—including ex-patients.

Visits in the homes of patients frequently provide more information for us and more opportunities for concrete help for the patient than a visit of the patient to the clinic would provide. While the contact person must be concerned with the patient and his medication, it is no longer a pill-dispensing role. Rather, the medication is the 'carrot' that opens the door. The visiting person may serve the patient in a number of ways ranging from home evaluation and counseling, to demonstration of home skills. Continuous communication and education with other agencies and individuals dealing with the patient is important in providing aftercare service.

In providing continuity of care for the patient, the policy of persistence and pursuit is a necessity. It often pays off in terms of the patient's functioning satisfactorily in the community.

Question:

I'm having trouble in selling any kind of group work in my rural community because I keep hearing that everyone knows each other and it would be impossible for a patient to be in a group with his next door neighbor. How do you work around this problem?

Miss Neufeld:

I've heard similar excuses from clients who say they don't have transportation; can't come to the clinic; wouldn't want so-and-so to bring them because then this person would know where they were going. I asked them for permission to contact the minister or whoever this significant 'other' is in the community, and subsequently, that person does bring them or sees to it that they have transportation. Frequently they find that their next door neighbor is in the group and sometimes they come and go together. The most difficult part is getting them there. Once they participate in the group, transportation doesn't seem to be a problem any more.

Comment:

In our rural county we have a supper club for discharged state-hospitalized patients at the Y.W.C.A. That's the way our group work started and it is now part of the resocialization treatment plan. Patients have come willingly, even with their neighbors as long as it wasn't the Community Mental Health Center where people could say that they were one of the community's mental health 'nuts.' In the groups, they have been able to talk about very personal problems.

Comment:

In our city we started a preschool nursery. The parents bring their children and then observe them. In addition, we run a parent discussion group with these families over a period of time.

Comment:

We have a volunteer church women's group who work with groups of mothers whose children are in the Headstart programs. Their younger pre-schoolers are now in a nursery school group—sort of a 'head start' Headstart program. The mothers' groups developed as their needs were identified; for example, sewing classes, nutrition, hair-styling. We meet in a downtown red brick mansion which looks more like an old, well-kept home than like the center of a mental health agency.

Comment:

In our community we utilize a known community agent as a co-group leader. We start out with a staff member and a community agent as trainer and trainee, and when the agent becomes competent, he carries the group alone. One such group experience was organized by a public health nurse and a former patient.

Comment:

Knowing that they were all former patients of the state hospital did not quell our apprehension about patients meeting their neighbors. At the first meeting we discussed what to call the group, thinking they would like to have other visible reasons for getting together for the sake of the community. When they decided to call themselves the 'Therapy Group,' we were surprised, and realized that some of the stigma is carried by the professional staff.

Comment:

I'm glad you mentioned that because I don't think our problem is with the client half as much as it is with the mental health people. We are often the ones who are afraid and feel insecure. We need to ask what the therapist's attitude about this problem is, and how skilled he is in handling it.

There's another concern involved here and that's the one of confidentiality. One of the first things the people in the community I work in brought up was that they were tired of being interviewed by teams of mental health professionals and spilling out personal problems. There may or may not be friends and relatives there and they felt that they really exposed themselves. Therefore, in the groups that I have, one of the things that I immediately deal with in the initial individual encounter and again in the group sessions, is the question of confidentiality, that is, the risk that anyone takes when he enters a group. I have learned that this is a primary concern. Some of our clients really don't care what other people hear, but they surely don't want it 'on paper.' One of the techniques that we have used in terms of putting things on paper is that we write the progress notes right in the group. We inform them that every two months, 'because of accreditation,' we have to record certain information in their chart. Then we ask what they want in their charts. Usually they'll give us a better progress note than we would have written ourselves. Because they dictate the notes and see them, they know exactly what's on record, and they don't seem to be as concerned about who else is going to see it.

Comment:

It seems to me the glaring omission in most community health centers is preparing the staff to learn something about the community the center is supposed to be serving. It also seems to me that a lot of the resistance is based on fear of the unknown. In my community, the center's staff members talk about safety on the streets and they are afraid to go into the community because the crime rate is so terribly high. They are afraid they are going to get mugged or raped, or something similar. To a certain extent, that is a realistic fear; in another sense, it's a red herring. They don't know the community and what they are going to have to do out there. Unless there's some kind of inservice going on in these centers, I don't think we are ever going to get at that resistance. There will be some few of us who are willing, interested, and want to take those risks, and find out what needs to be done; but others, particularly psychologists, psychiatrists, and social workers, seem to like to cling to that traditional model of seeing patients at the center—which is 'safe.' I really feel that's a fear of the unknown operating, and until we make that unknown known, fear will continue to exist.

Comment:

But—I'm not sure that's enough because even if an unknown is known, I think it takes time to feel comfortable with it, and that's the problem we have. You know—people choose where they want to spend their time and most of the therapists want to spend their time in their offices seeing their patients, and the only way they are going to learn to feel comfortable is by spending time in other areas, and we can't get them to do that.

Comment:

What we try to do is attach positive symbols to the Community Care Program, and now we are having trouble keeping people in the office because the prestige lies in the Community Care Program. So I think if we can give people a feeling that what they are doing is of primary importance to the agency, we can begin to motivate them to move out. As long as we keep the idea that prestige lies in the office with the big mahogany desks and all that other stuff, we are not going to get anyone out of the office.

Comment:

There are a couple of real differences as I see them in the whole idea of planning for pursuit. These are related to the distance that you have to go when you are working in a rural center, the time it takes, and the costs. You have to incorporate this in your budget and you have to incorporate it in your staff planning. How many people do you need—not for a 65,000 population but for the 6,500 miles a month or whatever it is of traveling distance. One of the things we have done to increase our manpower is to use the public health nurses, and they have been marvelous. In rural areas they know their people very, very well and they know the life situation of these people. I doubt if home visiting is financially any less expensive in the city. I know there was a study done at our Center and I wish I had taken a look at the breakdown on the figures, but for one of our nurses to make a home visit costs us an average of $52.00. So, I don't think it is just a matter of distance, but of salary and many other things.

There is a difference that I noticed in pursuit in the rural area versus pursuit in an urban area. In an urban area the large numbers of people concentrated in a small area makes pursuit more difficult than when you know that your patient lives somewhere near a farm road that's 20 miles away and you know exactly where that is, and where you are going to find him.

Comment:

I really don't have any experience in a rural area but I was very impressed with the fact that you pointed out that pursuit is essential, and also in presenting the difficulties that one encounters in working with chronically ill people. They are not always exciting and they are not always stimulating, but the challenges are different. We could really get caught up in a lot of rationalization as to who we should or should not pursue, based on expense and on location. I think the basic problem is that people do not want to participate in active pursuit. We have a catchment area of approximately 108,000 population. Our problems are minor in comparison to some of the things you are doing, but our people live close together; I don't know if we cover a 10-block square area, or maybe a 20-block square area, but our staff is reluctant to move out. We want them to move out. Now one would think that in that small an area one could pursue very easily. It's not a matter of expense and it really isn't that much time involved; people just don't want to go out. Also, people don't want to get bogged down with the chronic caseloads—they really don't.

Comments:

It took me three years to get a social worker to accompany me 50 miles to a home because I wanted him to see this person with whom I had worked for three years.

We have the same problem with somebody who lives three blocks away! It isn't the geographical area—it's the chronicity.

We can look at some of the reasons and how people handle these problems. We discharge staff as we recognize that they may not belong in our kind of setting.

I don't know that people are up to discharging staff for that reason, or whether there are some intermediate steps that have to be taken to help them out.

I think we would have to discharge about 70 percent of our staff if we were to do that—I'm serious, really. In my city, where everyone is supposedly sophisticated, many of our people have been trained or educated in a very traditional way. They are sophisticated in psychotherapy. They want to emulate the psychiatrist and the more traditional kinds of practice.

It has been our experience that only we nurses provide for continuity of care; for example, a patient will be admitted to the inpatient unit and very soon after admission, the outpatient therapist is assigned in order to develop a lasting relationship. When the patient is discharged, the outpatient therapist will talk to the patient prior to discharge and will make several appointments for the patient to return. Frequently, the patient doesn't show up. Well, I have to say that if it's a nurse involved, the nurse will be aggressive and move out to the home, but if it's a social worker, a psychologist or psychiatrist—(and we do have inter-disciplinary teams assigned in a rotating fashion)—what frequently happens is that the other professional will say, "I made about three or four appointments and the patient never showed up." Then about two or three months later, the patient comes back to our inpatient unit after the process of decompensation has started.

Question:

What about the services of the centers that are organized where the teams have lasting responsibility for a patient through all phases? Do you still have difficulty following the patients in the aftercare period?

Comment:

We have had experience with that type of organization. When a field worker in the community (a paraprofessional) picks up a patient, that worker continues to be the primary therapist in whatever service the client needs. For example, if the patient enters the inpatient service, his field worker continues to be the primary therapist, with medical back-up. When the patient re-enters the community, the field worker continues the care. The same is true in regard to outpatient treatment; there, the field worker is teamed with an outpatient psychiatric resident. If extensive services are needed, the resident and the field worker collaborate. The field worker visits the patient and the resident may visit also. All three always meet together when a patient is discharged. There are problems as this type of service is threatening to the residents. There are first-year residents in the inpatient unit and second-year residents in the outpatient units. When you have a field worker who is the primary therapist and he demands that the first-year resident listen to him and respect what he has to say—and, furthermore, back him up—that is threatening to the doctor in his role.

Comment:

We started out with that same system. When a person was admitted, regardless of service needed, he was assigned to a therapist who was responsible for him from then on. We found that as long as the person was an outpatient client, there was no problem; the therapist saw him once a week for an hour. As soon as the client came to the Day Care Program, the therapist didn't want the added responsibility for him 'when he got in trouble down there.' When he was admitted to the inpatient unit, the therapist again became so uncomfortable that the patient got lost.

Comment:
I don't have that problem with the field workers, as the concept of continuity of care has been built into their philosophy. The resistance comes from the professional level in the kind of collaborative work needed for field workers to function in their roles. The field worker has to negotiate with another system of which he is not a part; in other words, the outside therapist of a client in the inpatient unit has a critical problem in finding professionals there who are not only able but willing to negotiate.

The concept of continuity of care purports to provide a client with the most feasible continuous service. They may mean that one person is in contact with the client whenever and wherever he needs or seeks service. However, it may also mean that a client is turned over to the inpatient staff, and a new system assumes the primary responsibility for the client in that particular sector of services.

When other mental health professionals are unable or unwilling to implement the goals of the total program, the development of innovative modalities and services is retarded. The community mental health nurse is often faced with little choice but to continue to work alone. However, she cannot work alone without feeling powerless and futile in bringing about needed changes.

The Nurse Therapist as a Member of an Interdisciplinary Team

SHARON GEDAN, R.N., M.S.

The first community I lived in was on the south side of Chicago, Illinois. People living there who required psychiatric treatment were moved to a state institution, a foreboding brick building, miles from the city. Our community was thereby protected from emotional illness while families were disrupted and the patient was isolated and institutionalized.

In college, I learned to nurse psychiatric patients in a small Los Angeles community hospital. Unlike the Chicago institution, the buildings were surrounded by trees and gardens, and the staff took pride in giving personalized care. Nonetheless, patients were still isolated from the community and were still institutionalized.

Today, as a clinical specialist, I practice in Hawaii's Straub Clinic. Our clinic building is located in central Honolulu. However, patients I nurse live throughout the Hawaiian Islands. Depending on their nursing needs, I may see them in the clinic, home, school, a general hospital, or a psychiatric unit.

Psychiatric treatment methods have changed a great deal, and psychiatric nurses are being offered opportunities for greater responsibility in patient care. However, so much change has occurred that the nurse's place in treatment has often been unclear. At the Straub Clinic, we have developed a role which is satisfying to the psychiatric nurse, her co-workers, and her patients. Since psychiatric nurses throughout the country are in the process of developing useful treatment roles, an exploration of the work being done by our team may be useful.

THE INTERDISCIPLINARY TEAM

The successful functioning of our team is influenced by the kind of people we are, the expectations we have of one another, and the complementary relationships we have developed. Our psychiatrist is a competent therapist who delegates responsibility for patient care and does not infringe on the freedom of the psychologist. The psychologist, skilled in therapy and testing, seeks the assistance of the psychiatrist for medical problems and offers us guidance with psychological techniques. Both men are comfortable sharing the responsibility for patient care with a nurse so that I am encouraged to take an active part in therapy.

The factor which is most important to me is that I am recognized as a professional person whose work is respected. I spend my time doing work that I like and in which I have specialized training. Supervision is available to me as I need it, and I am continually encouraged to be a creative and responsible therapist.

To understand how we function, I would like to describe the community we serve and the services we offer. I will elaborate the therapeutic approach I use, and describe three nursing treatment modalities which our team finds effective.

Hawaii is composed of six major inhabited islands. There is a myth that Hawaii is an island paradise and, in fact, our weather is beautiful and relatively unchanging. But we have most of the "big city problems" found in other communities. We have a cosmopolitan population of which the vast majority is Oriental. As a Caucasian, I am unique in the United States: I am a member of a minority group.

The Hawaiian Islands have been a state since August 21, 1959. It is considered a democratic state where the economy is marked by heavy expenditures from the military, agriculture, and tourism, and where the cost of living and taxes are among the highest in the nation. People come to Hawaii for many reasons. Tourists come to play and sometimes for a "magic rest cure;" coeds come for their first fling at freedom; "hippies" come to find a land of love, and surfers come to ride the big waves; military families come on rest and recreation; movie companies come on location; and the rich elderly come for retirement. All of these factors affect our patient population.

Services Provided

Our psychiatric treatment facilities include a state hospital, which is primarily a residence for chronic patients; an acute unit located in a general hospital, and an intermediate treatment unit. Thirty psychiatrists practice in our

Table 1.

SERVICES PROVIDED

	Psychiatrist	Psychologist	Nurse
Individual Psychotherapy	X	X	
Group Psychotherapy	X	X	X
Initial Consultation	X	X	
Psychiatric Nurse Counseling			X
Psychological Testing		X	
Family Therapy	X		
Crisis Intervention	X	X	X
Sensitivity Training			X
Social Evaluation			
Evaluation of Children		X	
Treatment of Children		X	
Consultation to Community Agencies	X	X	X
Research on treatment of Psychosomatic Illness	X	X	X
Consultation to Hospital Specialty Units	X		X
Counseling of family Members	X	X	
Assistance with Placement			
Home Visits	X		X
Consultation to all other Straub Clinic Departments	X	X	X

state with approximately forty clinical psychologists and five clinical specialists in psychiatric nursing.

The Straub Clinic is a private partnership of 72 doctors serving in all medical specialties. Our department of psychiatry, psychology, and family relations offers a wide variety of services. A summary of what is currently available is found in Table 1. We schedule our services in keeping with our belief that patients need to maintain a normal routine. The department is open three evenings a week and every Saturday and two psychotherapy groups meet during lunch hour. Future plans include additional staff, an inpatient unit, continued research, and a more extensive consultative service.

One of our objectives is to insure efficient delivery of services to patients, and to accomplish this end, good working relationships among our staff are essential. Each of us expects and receives the support of his co-workers. The psychologist is welcomed by the psychiatrist as an equal, and the limits of the nurse's participation are set only by her education and ability. Although there has been controversy in our community about the jurisdiction of psychiatrists and psychologists, this is not an issue in our department.

We have established a climate in which we talk about patients and ourselves, and we are able to comment on what we see as each other's strengths and weaknesses. The nurse's comments are valued and utilized which is a significant morale factor. We talk during our weekly staff lunch, during informal supervision, and in consultation and in treatment sessions with more than one therapist. Lambertsen expresses what we have found: "It is the perogative of the practitioners of the profession to define the core of professional service. Related groups are concerned, but the final determination of the professional mission is the right and responsibility of the practitioner."

My particular interest is co-leading psychotherapeutic groups. In the past year and a half, I have co-led seven groups and have led one group for obese patients. The benefits of two therapists for group therapy has been examined in psychiatric literature and will not be reviewed here. In our particular groups, we found that patients will often prefer to talk in groups with the nurse, who is seen as less of an authority figure than the doctor, and patients will have greater opportunity to work through parental conflicts with both a male and female therapist. An example of this occurred in a recent group session:

N., a depressed secretary, began talking about how upset she felt. After the doctor expressed interest in learning more about her pain, she exploded in an hysterical tirade, accusing the doctor of hating her and 'always hating' her. The doctor then suggested to the patient that she talk with me, and by moving his chair and remaining silent, he responded to N.'s need for distance from him. In the group's presence, he then acted as a consultant to me, suggesting areas for me to explore with her and assisting with interpretations. At the end of the session, N. was able to talk with him about how angry and afraid of him she had been. This is perhaps one example of what has been described as the complementary work of psychiatrist and nurse-therapist.[3]

My contact with group patients is not limited to group therapy sessions. I see any group patient who experiences a crisis between sessions. Crisis offers opportunity for significant movement in therapy. When it is possible for a therapist to be with the patient when his emotional wound is open, valuable diagnostic material can be obtained, this is better than relying on the often distorted recollections of the patient. The nurse, whose schedule is the most flexible in our setting, is often the only team member available to be with the patient at that critical time.

THERAPEUTIC APPROACH

Nurses assist patients during times of intense suffering. Our basic education includes caring for persons in pain, at times of emergency, during childbirth, and at death. There is a common quality to all human suffering, and nursing experience prepares us to recognize emotional suffering in the psychiatric patient. Response to the patient's suffering is the basic therapeutic approach we use. An effective response brings about an emotional involvement between the patient and the nurse-therapist. A relationship is thereby initiated in which the patient can experiment with new ways of feeling, acting, and being.

The response I make to patients is a combination of caring and confrontation in something like an 80 to 20 percent ratio. The patient is experiencing some kind of emotional pain, and caring is the human involvement which makes the pain bearable, encourages trust, and allows for confrontation. Confrontation is necessary because the patient is not aware of his ineffective manner of meeting his needs. In order to change, he has to become aware of what he is doing, and this information needs to reach his awareness with enough impact to promote change.

Psychiatric nurses recognize the importance of assisting patients with "here and now" problems. The therapeutic approach I am describing expands the meaning of here and now to include all that occurs between the patient and therapist in the present. It is necessary to understand and accept "the vital importance of the immediate, the present, the whole, not exclude perspective, but to establish a central point to which that perspective can be readily related." The following example illustrates emphasis on the patient's present experience:

M. was referred to our department for treatment of persistent migraine headaches. As she entered my office, tears welled up in her eyes, she held them back with her hand, and began to talk immediately as she seated herself. I commented on her struggle not to cry. She ignored my comment and began to say she didn't know what to do about an impossible situation in her life. I reacted again to her tears and to her brushing off my invitation to cry. By focusing on the present, I communicated to her that regardless of the impossible situation at home, something painful was happening to her in my office.

Through this discussion we learned a great deal about the kind of person she is. An understanding of herself was of far greater value during our therapeutic work together than a direct discussion of situations in her life.

The nursing intervention with M.'s feelings is of additional interest because it demonstrates another aspect of our therapeutic approach—the expression of affect. Painful emotions are to be shared during the therapy session. Complete expression is demanded by the therapist so that feelings are shared and not merely talked about. Emotional illness is, after all, a form of human suffering which cannot be relieved by discussion and intellectual understanding alone.

Involvement of the nurse-therapist is essential to our approach. The use of self as a therapeutic tool has long been recognized in nursing. Orlando defined the nurse's own reaction as an essential element of the nursing process: "This reaction consists of three aspects: 1) perceptions of the patient's behavior, 2) the thoughts stimulated by the perceptions, and 3) feelings in response to these perceptions and thoughts."[4] In nursing therapy, these three elements of the nurse' reaction are expertly utilized in response to the patient.

TREATMENT MODALITIES

The way the nurse structures her time with patients should depend on the patient's immediate difficulty and the overall treatment plan established with his doctor. We have overwhelming evidence that traditional psychiatric therapies are inefficient and we can predict that, with our present national priorities, we will never have sufficient professional mental health workers. The psychiatric nursing specialist who is less hampered by tradition than members of other disciplines, must participate in new treatment forms.

One treatment form found effective is what we call the "minimarathon." During a twelve-month period, five patients have been treated with this technique. Patients are referred on an emergency basis to one of our doctors by a general practitioner on an island without an adequate psychiatric facility. Patients are then seen for a diagnostic consultation by one of our doctors, a conference is held with the doctor, the patient, and the nurse, and the immediate therapeutic goal is determined. I then work with the patient in an intensive marathon until the goal is accomplished. In each case thus far, hospitalization was avoided and the patient returned to his family and work with little disruption to his normal routine. The minimarathon at Straub closely follows the principles of brief psychotherapy as described by Stroker which are to "apply techniques which aid in the resolution of temporary crises and permit further independence and ego growth to continue unaided." An example follows:

Mrs. K., a Hawaiian-Japanese housewife from the island of Kauai, was the first patient with whom we worked in a minimarathon. She was treated in a four-hour marathon with a one-hour follow-up the following day. Her diagnosis was an acute anxiety reaction, exhibited primarily by severe and constant shaking of her legs. She initiated our session by stating she was told by our psychologist that she needed to learn how to express her anger. We began our work with her reaction to our psychologist's statement and quickly realized that she was equating thoughts and feelings, and also that she had a distorted view of anger. In her mind, anger equalled violence. At one point, Mrs. K didn't like a comment made to her and we learned how she converted her irritation to physical symptoms. She clearly described a burning sensation in her feet which proceeded up her legs, felt like butterflies in her stomach, rose into her neck, and ended with a nauseating lump in her throat. When she verbalized her anger, physical conversions of her feelings subsided. As she worked, I pointed out to her that we were gaining an understanding of her symptoms and that she had a lot of work to do on her own. Mrs. K returned to the care of her physician and has made two phone calls to the clinic for information and reassurance since that time. Her symptoms have subsided and her marital relationship, previously impaired, has improved.

A second treatment method, the home visit, is familiar in nursing but can be further adapted to accomplish specific psychiatric goals:

Home visits to Miss S were initiated on a biweekly basis to enable early discharge from the psychiatric hospital and to prevent rehospitalization. Miss S has a history of severe depression, life-threatening weight loss, and poor insight. Her needs are beyond the skills of the public health nurses in our community. In the past, she had disappeared between hospitalizations and had rapidly deteriorated. At the present time, a non-threatening relationship with the nurse therapist is being utilized to encourage appropriate problem-saving.

The third treatment innovation we are using is preparation for group therapy. We no longer need documentation to recognize group therapy as an efficient treatment method to assist larger numbers of patients while instituting less dependence on the therapist. Our team is currently treating eight groups of eight patients each. We have found that patients can benefit from group therapy more quickly and are more likely to remain in group treatment if they are "nursed into the group." The patients are seen by a doctor in consultation and when group therapy is selected as the treatment of choice, they are referred to the nurse for preparation for group therapy. They are seen individually to work through any initial resistances to treatment and to acquaint them with our treatment approach. Patients often feel more comfortable working with a nurse, begin to trust her as someone who will support them, and can therefore participate more openly in the group. A sample of this approach follows:

Mr. and Mrs. P were referred to a group for treatment of his depressive reaction and her psychosomatic illness. Our psychologist noted that Mrs. P was preoccupied with somatic complaints, and that the couple would probably resist, as they had in the past, any attempt to influence their emotional difficulties. Mrs. P had had a brief experience in an inpatient therapy group which she found painful and frightening. In a series of nursing interviews, this initial resistance was worked through and the couple were introduced to each other as "emotional people." They were then able to begin group treatment.

Each of these techniques results in less expense to the patient, better use of the psychiatrist or psychologist's skill, and additional therapy time which might not otherwise have been available. These treatment forms were developed in response to particular needs in our community but could be applied in other settings.

SUMMARY

At the Straub Clinic, an interdisciplinary psychiatric team assists patients who live throughout the Hawaiian Islands. A clinical specialist in psychiatric nursing has developed a useful and satisfying role on this team. The nurse therapist's role includes preparing patients for treatment, supporting and sustaining them during treatment, assisting patients directly through nursing therapy, and continually seeking more effective ways of caring for and comforting patients in emotional pain.

REFERENCES

1. Lambertson, E.C. Education for nursing leadership. Philadelphia, J.B. Lippincott Co., 1958, p. 49.
2. Mellow, J. Nursing therapy Amer. J. Nurs., 11:2365, November, 1968.
3. Kempler, W. Experiental Family Therapy. Int. J. Group Psychother., 15:57, January, 1965.
4. Orlando, I.J. The dynamic nurse-patient relationship: function, process and principles. New York, G.P. Putnam's Sons, 1961, p. 40.
5. Straker, M. Brief psychotherapy in an outpatient clinic: evolution and evaluation, Amer. J. Psychiat., 124:1219-26, March, 1968.

DISCUSSION

Question:

Before you started your paper, you mentioned the 48-hour marathon of staff. Would you elaborate why that came about?

Mrs. Gedan:

I think all of us are committed to therapy as a human experience. Each one of us sees this. I see my life and my involvement as a human experience, not as something that can be learned from textbooks. It's something you have to go through together; something that has to do with being a human being. It's only when you go through this experience that you develop empathy. We have a therapist who believed as we do, and he is an expert at guiding people in this type of experiential therapy.

We began to establish this atmosphere when we first opened our department. The three members of our team and nine other therapists in the community came together for a weekend and we had a 48-hour marathon where our roles of nurses or psychologists were forgotten. We got together on the level of "just people," which increased awareness of the kind of person each of us are—what our strengths are, what our weaknesses are, the kinds of things that we are afraid of, and what we have to offer, of our individual hangups in working with patients. We have continued this group twice a year since that time, with our spouses, when they want to come, and this has made a big difference in getting the kind of support we need from each other.

Question:

Could you elaborate a little bit more on what you mean by nursing therapy?

Mrs. Gedan:

I always assume that my patient is in pain because of the ineffective way he is caring for his needs. It is my responsibility to listen to him, observe him, and pick up what it is that he is doing that is inefficient, and confront him with that. At the same time, I know that he has developed this inefficient way of handling his needs for a very good reason. I know that becoming aware of what he is doing is a very painful experience, about which I have a lot of feeling. My responsibility is twofold: to learn more about him and to respond to his pain as it unfolds, and to confront him with his inefficient behavior. I might say that our sessions are extremely active. Patients do not "chat;" they do not discuss; they come in and everyone in the room knows that we're all there because suffering is evident. We share that suffering and we don't want just to talk to him about the situation. There's a lot of yelling, swearing, crying and screaming, and, as a result, a great deal of comfort is given to our patients. We find this very effective.

The goal of all of our work with patients is to help them cope with life more effectively. We continually expect all of our patients to be actively involved in their treatment and show significant change.

Question:

What background do you consider necessary for the nurse therapist?

Mrs. Gedan:

What was necessary for me but not necessarily true of anyone else, was graduate education and learning about psychiatric theory. Following this, I had the opportunity to work as a clinical specialist in an acute psychiatric unit with few tools except myself. I worked for three years on an acute unit in Hawaii and I didn't allow the staff to lock patients up or use restraints. I insisted that we all use ourselves as therapeutic tools; that's where I learned the most.

I discussed in my paper that I think what nurses have to offer is our familiarity with human suffering because, if you have supported a woman in labor, or a family when they've had a member with a terminal illness, or a mother when her baby is stillborn, you know what suffering is. With a psychiatric patient, the behavior you observe is different—you pick up that quality that is common to human suffering, and that's what we, as nurses, respond to intuitively.

Question:

I think the system you have is great, but in a developing community mental health center such as the one in which I work, the staff are not as experienced as most of us at this table or have the kinds of education most of us have had; we're beginning with a first-level nurse. Of the things that you pointed out, which one of these skills do you think we can focus on?

Mrs. Gedan:

You've got to begin *before* your first-level nurse. One has to have a certain amount of self-confidence and self-assurance before one can build up either technical or professional skills. I think one begins by recruiting a person with those personal qualifications into nursing in the first place, and we need to revamp our educational system.

When I consult with first-level nurses in a community and I tell them, "I haven't the slightest idea what your clients need—spend some time with the patients and see what you can identify. Each one of you is different, each one of you has something to offer." And you also have to tell them, "You don't have to be a supernurse the first time you talk with a patient. You don't have to cure him; go spend several hours with one patient and find out what you have to offer him. And if you believe you have something to offer, then you do—you really do."

Many times I give concrete suggestions to students. When I'm anxious and frightened about the students, I sometimes go and spend time with them but I think it is disrespectful to nurses to believe that they can't function individually. I might say, "If you want some help from me, I am willing to give it to you."

Comment:

You have to know something first before you can be creative; once you have information, you can build. On the other hand, if you give too much direction—make them dependent on you—there is difficulty in learning to be creative. The problem isn't what the student comes with, it's our inability to build on it, to appreciate it, to capitalize on it—and I'm trying to avoid the word "teach" but rather, living-learning kind of situation. I wish students would be more uproarish and do more stuff because that's going to be our salvation.

Comment:

We were feeling the same kind of struggle in creating our own role—a sort of birth agony. We are now questioning how to help the students, the paraprofessionals, new staff or whatever they are. Can we prepare them so that they're going to have an easier time, perhaps spare them some of the agony? The problem with that is you can't tell someone because being a different person, they're going to have a different experience anyway. However, when people start to develop and grow and you see a ruddy path ahead, whether or not you're going to let them go ahead and experience it, will depend on how high the risk is. If someone is going to walk on the high wall and you know that there's a brick loose, and there's a chance of their falling, you've got to stop them, whereas if it's a matter of stumbling over a couple of obstacles here and there, you're inclined to let them stumble. How much you can just sit back and allow people to learn those things themselves and how much you need to guide, assist, support, and instruct has to be balanced. You can't prevent people from taking some hard knocks and having some difficulties entering your system.

Comment:

In my graduate program, it took me two years to fight for a meaningful clinical experience. This struggle took me to nursing faculty and nursing administration. I had to get help and backing from a psychiatrist so that I could accomplish my goal. I now work in a child psychiatric hospital which is part of a university. They have a training program for psychiatric residents and a program for social workers. It functions from a traditional psychoanalytic orientation; the child belongs to the medical therapist, the parents to the social worker, the nurse tends the ward. No one works with the entire family, in the home, in the community, either for prevention, treatment or aftercare. It took me a year to become accepted as a nursing clinical specialist in the hospital before I dared bring other nurses out in the community.

I've had some success; the nurses are now involved in total family therapy, preventive work, and follow-up. We have become active, contributing team members not just passively sitting by taking orders. In order to make home visits with the entire family, nurses are able to have flexible hours, 1:00 P.M.-10:00 P.M. or 2:00 P.M.- 12:00 A.M., depending on the needs. The other disciplines all jumped on the bandwagon regarding home visits but they do not go out themselves. Therefore, my goal is to get more nurses involved in this but I have to work through the nurse's fears—"I don't know what to do or how to do it."

At times it is painful and discouraging to buck the system. I have lost friends because they've given up trying to fight; they moved out to places where they are accepted. I want to continue because there is a vast number of people who need this service. If I move out the water will cover it over. I gradually want to lose my position once I get those nurses doing their thing—getting their work fully accepted as part of the system in the hospital. I've only worked with nurses in one section; there are two other wards operating as before. A small group of us tried to constructively devise a plan for the hospital, to become more responsive to the needs of the community. We outlined what we should be doing. It was taken out of our hands, put up into the hierarchial system—to the administrative officers. It's been underground for a year, nothing has been done, no reports issued. Those of us who are out in the community know what's going on. But we had to push forward and then we were pushed out.

Mrs. Gedan:

I've had a similar experience for over three years, "doing my thing," arguing, struggling, demonstrating, and proving. I've reached a point where I'm convinced that it was meeting my needs at that time or I wouldn't have been there. One thing that was useful to me, in addition to short-term goals, was to set long-range goals. I estimated that it would take 10 years to work through some of the problems we had with the public health nurses working with psychiatric patients in the community. If you expect to do everything in three years, you're bound to get frustrated.

Comment:

All of us working with new people need to sit down with them and help them to identify for themselves the "know-how" that they have. Nurses often have trouble with this; they need to be encouraged to deal with their fear about using this "know-how." Most nurses can be very effective with patients in some way. If they make a mistake, it's not written in stone; someone can help them correct this.

STAFF DEVELOPMENT

Historically, nurses have sought professional advancement by way of routes leading to positions of administrator and teacher so that they will receive increased recognition, status, and remuneration. A recent trend to refocus on the patient and his experience, has led some agencies to reorganize nursing practice offering the "bedside" nurse upward mobility. The emergence and recognition of the nurse clinical specialist has additionally opened channels for a nurse not only to rise in the ranks but to receive satisfaction for doing well what she knows and wants to do. Most recently, some psychiatric-mental health clinicians who have experienced in their practice how various systems block the way to better patient care, have accepted administrative and teaching positions in order to have direct access to locus of power and thus bring about needed change in the training and utilization of community mental health personnel and to insure meaningful and continuous care of patients.

In order to increase community mental health manpower and to further develop existing manpower, continuous education—including new types of training—is required so that the process of role expansion can move in new directions. The need for imaginative and creative methods of recruiting, training, retaining, and utilization of manpower, particularly paraprofessional staff from the local neighborhoods is critical. In sustaining paraprofessionals in their work experience, supportive services are of major importance. Collaborative efforts between the professional, paraprofessional, and client are essential to the development of relevant, responsive services.

Perhaps the most interesting discoveries made by mental health workers have been that neighborhood people know the neighborhood best and, since it is necessary to service clients in a unified team approach, the training of personnel needs to be combined and carried out in a unified manner.

This chapter describes nurses' influence on the philosophy of particular clinical programs, on role designation, and on patterns of training and care. Community mental health nurses work within a socio-psychiatric orientation, integrating intrapsychic, interpersonal, social, and cultural phenomena. They are actively seeking ways to focus on mental health instead of on mental illness by identifying and promoting clients' reserves and strengths, which are the foundation of mental health.

Expanding the community mental health nurse's role as a member of the tradition-oriented psychiatric team requires planning, strategy, negotiation, and collaboration with other professionals, paraprofessionals, and particularly with clients and with members of the community. The strategies cited include informing others about psychiatric nursing education and practice; learning and appreciating the value systems and problems of the clients and the community; and anticipating the consequences of role changes in a shifting environment. While moving in the direction of a more coordinated interdependent relationship with other professionals in which the nursing personnel are prepared to assume responsibility for clinical practice and to share in the decision-making, nurses have encountered "skepticism, ridicule, bias, good-natured disbelief, and resistance" but, also, "tremendous positive support."

The training experts, whose papers follow, describe the nurse as a planner, designer, and trainer in staff development programs for groups of people with heterogeneous backgrounds. Basic assumptions underlying the use of combined training programs are that each individual has a valuable contribution to make to the group, and that training serves to maximize the potential of each individual. Training methods reflect the belief that training, rather than telling people *what* to think, teaches them *how* to think, how to conceptualize and identify a problem and how to arrive at the best way of solving it.

Learning takes place experientially in a variety of ways, particularly through group process, sensitivity training, cross-cultural confrontation, and seminars. These experiences help staff develop questioning attitudes and the expectation of being heard, and open a much needed "two-way learning street" between trainer and trainee. Moreover, the interrelated training and utilization of paraprofessional staff has led to a re-examination of the perceptions and value systems of all involved and has led to personal growth in staff members. Training programs have further resulted in the sharing of power and in giving the paraprofessional control over his destiny. The paraprofessional is not merely a link in bridging the manpower gap, but is a member of a group that can broaden and improve services because of its ability to bring out the strengths of clients and the community.

Generally the advanced formal educational system has been used to determine the entry and upward mobility of mental health practitioners. Some conferees believe it is necessary to change the system to allow experience to be one basis for employment and upward mobility. One conferee pointed out; "This is nothing new—this concept was advantageous in the past; the problem was that many clinical agencies did not want to assume the responsibility of making judgments about the abilities of their workers and therefore turned this responsibility over to academia."

Emerging Issues in Training for Community Mental Health Nursing

NANCY H. FRENCH, R.N., M.S.

Training for practice in community mental health nursing demands clarity of purpose not only with regard to function but also to one's own philosophies of psychiatric nursing, mental health, education and, most broadly, life itself. These philosophies must then be compared with those of the institution or insititutions where the training will occur. It must be stressed that a statement of philosophy for a training program must be more than an intellectual exercise and cannot be seen as one-dimensional. It should also be noted that individual and institutional philosophy is not static so that a review of this philosophy for training must be ongoing. While it may seem to be a formidable task, the success of training programs rests on the foundation provided by these philosophies.[1, 2] The importance of these bases is highlighted by two definitions of philosophy: (1) "a system of principles for guidance in practical affairs; and (2) "a system of values by which one lives."[3, 4]

One example of opposing educational philosophies relevant to current training programs in community mental health nursing is based on: (1) "whether the individual has responsibility for improvement of social conditions."[5] The first emphasizes adjustment to and fitting into the system while the second focuses on developing the ability of critical analysis and then serving as a change agent for individual function or for the system as a whole.[6] While all of us responsible for the development of training programs might feel we strongly subscribe to the second principle, how often are we building program objectives and experiences on the first? Questions such as this become critically significant as we plan training programs for nursing personnel, both professional and nonprofessional, to prepare them to practice in community mental health. One important means of providing opportunity for implementation of analysis and change agents is to train *together* those people who will be working together.

At the present time we should examine both the changing role for nursing personnel, as we move into more active involvement in prevention, and the changes in philosophy that may be required to adequately train for this new focus. If we continue to accept the philosophy and assumptions found in the statement on psychiatric nursing practice published by the American Nurses' Association, we will seriously limit the potential effectiveness of community mental health nursing.[7] In the section on philosophy and assumptions there is a focus on pathology that is exemplified by one particular statement: "Psychiatric nursing is a service to people who are affected by pathological thought processes."[8] Statements relating to prevention also begin with the patient as a base. This perpetuates a concentration on the prevention of mental illness rather than on the promotion of mental health since it is easily translated at the action level into looking at communities and individuals from the point of view of identifying pathology and weakness in which we intervene, rather than from a perspective of identification and promotion of strengths which are the foundation of mental health.

As you may have noted, I have thus far consistently talked of training for community mental health nursing and the joint training of all levels of nursing personnel. The stress is purposeful and important as a philosophical basis for training. As we move from the academic environment, where the primary emphasis is on the development of nurses and their professional identity, to the service environment, we must also shift our emphasis in training to a primary focus on the provision of creative prevention, treatment, and rehabilitation services. This shift requires that we train people together for the work that must be done. It must not be assumed that the professional has more knowledge and skills in all areas. Rather, we assume that the professional brings to the job certain knowledge and skills which are needed by the nonprofessional, and that the community person has life experience and knowledge of the community he comes from. By training the groups separately, both will lose valuable data and knowledge. If the professional nurses and other professionals along with the nonprofessionals, can debate with one another and try out, through role-playing and other exercises, many ways of handling the same problem or issue, then, when they are working together, they are more likely to be able to capitalize on one another's strengths.

In the service setting it is important to begin with the basic assumption that everyone has an important contribution to make to the mental health team and that training is provided to maximize the potential of each individual and group so that interest, creativity, skills and each person's capacity can be fostered and capitalized on. Thus training, rather than teaching people *what* to think, becomes a means to teach staff how to think, *how* to conceptualize a problem, and how to arrive at the best way of solving it. This does not mean that specific skill training is underemphasized; it does mean that the skill training must not only be "this is the way we do things here," but also "this is why, at the moment, we have chosen to do things this way." When people are trained with this philosophy and have a basic questioning attitude it may mean that we in leadership positions will have many uncomfortable moments both during the training and later, when individuals have begun to work as staff members.

Staff who complete such a program will challenge leadership to listen to their point of view and they will expect to be heard. For example, recently a staff group challenged me on a form of teaching I was using in an ongoing program on one of the units at the Connecticut Mental Health Center. When they felt I was not fully listening to them, they worked together on a document presenting not only their points of view but their ideas on how our sessions should be conducted. Their action was a responsible one and their proposal was accepted after negotiation with only minor modifications. I was gratified at their action because they demonstrated the capacity to be creative and constructive in their criticism rather than "acting out" by decreasing their attendance at class or participating less when they were present. A combination of psychiatric aides and graduate nurses who had been trained together comprised the group who jointly presented their thinking to me. Obviously, part of what they had learned in their joint training sessions was how to work together as a group.

Still another reason we should examine the training together of nursing personnel who will be working together, is that if, in community mental health, we accept the idea that interlocking partnerships are necessary between the community and the hospital, and between nursing and other professionals, then we cannot stop the partnership line when we reach the nonprofessional who works in nursing service. As more and more bright, capable community people are attracted to work as psychiatric aides (in some places called mental health workers) we must look at what they have to teach us as well as deciding what skill training they will need. It is these community people who often can be of great value to us in questioning our practice as it is related to the needs of their neighborhood, particularly in the inner city environment. They can help us broaden our scope of understanding about how we determine when someone needs traditional psychiatric services and when other types of services might be more effective. We cannot overlook the tremendous importance of the psychiatric aide or mental health worker in extending the volume and quality of services offered by community mental health centers. Now let us look at the process by which training has been implemented at the Connecticut Mental Health Center (CMHC).

THE SETTING

The CMHC is an institution that has been established as a joint endeavor between the State of Connecticut and Yale University. All senior professional staff are employed by Yale and serve as active teaching faculty. Most staff social workers and all nursing personnel (beginning at the head nurse level) are Civil Service employees.

The Yale University School of Nursing entered the joint endeavor convinced that the school and the clinical facility both would benefit by the integration of nursing service and nursing education. The contract provided for joint appointments of a director, two associate directors and nine clinical specialists for nursing service. These faculty members are responsible for working with members of other disciplines in the planning of and training for mental health services offered by specific units and by the total institution.

The Center was conceived, money was appropriated by the state legislature, and the architectural design was virtually completed before President Kennedy delivered his address on mental illness and mental retardation in 1963.[9] This has had great implications for the programs established at the CMHC, because the philosophy on which it was established called for an institution which would be a model treatment facility for the total state of Connecticut, as well as a training and research facility for the Yale University School of Medicine. Thus when President Kennedy called for a "bold new approach" with a focus on prevention and comprehensive community care central to new mental health programs; it seemed impossible for the new philosophy to be totally implemented. The Center was regionalized to service New Haven and 13 surrounding suburban towns. This meant the total population to be serviced was approximately 400,000–200,000 more than the catchment areas allowed by NIMH criteria. With 83 beds and 40 day hospital spaces the Center could not meet the treatment needs of this population, and preventive work was even more overwhelming. (Major portions of the treatment needs of the area are still met by a large state hospital 25 miles from New Haven.) In addition, the psychiatric residency training program in the Yale Department of Psychiatry, was traditional and gave little emphasis to prevention.

A partial solution to this problem was accomplished through the establishment of one division which would be responsible for a catchment area with 75,000 people. Two neighborhoods were included in that catchment, one an inner city neighborhood in the midst of marked social transition, the other a contiguous town with a range of social classes two through five.[10] This service, called the Hill-West Haven Unit, was designed to offer comprehensive mental health services. It was charged with the responsibility not only to implement innovative programs but to study these programs in terms of the delivery of services and aspects of community control. The rest of the Center has the following units: inpatient, outpatient, emergency treatment (crisis intervention with a patient stay of three to five days with 30-day follow-up as outpatients), inpatient research, day hospital, and an education and consultation division. There has been tension present in relation to the philosophy and approach since the beginning of clinical planning; these were the result of differing expectations of the state, the Yale School of Medicine, the Yale School of Nursing, and the community itself. However, as stated by Dr. G.L. Klerman, the former director of the Center: "The efforts to cope with the problems of New Haven are not just the struggles of a particular mental health center in a particular city. Rather, they typify the exploratory approach needed by any community mental health center to deal with the urban problems in any city."[11] The establishment of training programs for nursing personnel was strongly effected by the various philosophies, objectives, and purposes—not only of individual units but of the larger institutions.

THE PLANNING YEAR

The planning year was used by the director of nursing and one assistant director to establish a foundation for an active, collaborative, expandable role for nursing personnel within the psychiatric team. The close working relationship between the director and assistant director was a major factor in the success we obtained in establishing both a creative role for nursing personnel in the Center and the training program itself. While the director held primary responsibility for nursing leadership in program development, the assistant director was responsible for the development of training programs; there was much sharing of responsibility in strategy, planning, and negotiations with others. From the beginning, both considered training a top priority and often focused on that priority in the planning group established. That group included the clinical director, the acting directors of social work and psychology, several chiefs of clinical units, and the director and assistant director of nursing.

The strategies used by the nursing leaders were as follows: (1) opportunities were sought to inform those assembled of trends in psychiatric nursing education and service; (2) attempts were made to anticipate (with others) the potential consequences of role changes in nursing, bearing in mind that nursing was a part of a role system. For example, we were attempting to move away from a strict medical model where the doctor prescribes treatment and the nurse carries out orders; we wanted to move in the direction of a more coordinated interdependent relationship in which nursing personnel would be prepared to assume responsibility for clinical practice and share in decision making; (3) through active participation in discussions, attempts were also made to influence the philosophy of clinical programs, the patterns of care, the role designations; and, where possible, attitudes toward nursing so that the way could be opened for experimentation and change.

Resistance, skepticism, bias, ridicule, good natured disbelief, and at times personal ambiguity and anxiety were encountered by the nurse leaders; but there were also positive supporting forces. The discussions were most helpful in forcing them to become clearer in their own conceptions and at the end of this phase, a preservice education program was designed and presented as a method for preparing nursing personnel to function in this highly diverse organization. The program included core content, necessary for practice on all units, with additional content and change in methods built in so that staff would be specifically prepared to work on a particular unit. This flexibility proved itself in a developing freedom for nursing to design and implement certain forms of practice.

On the inpatient and day hospital services, emphasis was on the therapeutic community and small groups. From the emergency treatment unit, with its emphasis on crisis intervention, the training program focused on individual work. For the Hill-West Haven Unit, nursing personnel had to be trained not only for inpatient and day hospital care but also for community involvement and field service programs including case finding, home treatment, and close interagency work. While a community activities division (devoted fully to preventive services) was established only in the past two years, preventive aspects of mental health had been woven throughout the original preservice programs. When it was formed, the Community Activities Division staff came primarily from existing nursing staff in the Institution.

THE PRESERVICE PROGRAM

The principles on which the preservice program was based were set forth in the CMHC "Position Paper on Staffing," presented to the Commissioner of Mental Health and his staff in November, 1965. Specifically in relation to preservice and later continuing inservice education programs it stated, ". . . we look forward to strengthing our nursing practice and providing depth in trained people. Our goal will be to upgrade the level of competence of all nursing personnel, maximize the potential of the most willing and achieve a high level of staff development to the end that the patient receives the best possible services."

The major broad objective and justification for the preservice training program was that it would establish organized treatment teams so that when patients were admitted to each service they would be received into an organized social system, ready to begin treatment without a preservice program. Where all levels of nursing personnel were trained together, patients would have been admitted into an unstable environment because personnel from various backgrounds would not have had an opportunity to build any unified basic philosophy of patient care. The specific rolls of members of the nursing staff were ultimately planned and developed by the senior leadership team of each service.

As the director and assistant director interviewed people applying for positions in nursing, it became very clear that a preservice program would be essential since few applicants were prepared to work in the setting. Further support for the design of a preservice program was gained from recommendations by the National League for Nursing that nursing personnel should have a period preceding service obligations that would be devoted to preparation for their work roles in an institution. We were in a particularly advantageous position to offer such a program since we were starting with a completely new staff in a new mental health center, and all staff for any given unit could be hired for a three-month training period preceding the opening of the service to which they were assigned.

In the clinical planning group, many questions were raised during the preliminary discussion of the need for a preservice training period. The service chiefs in particular wondered if the training couldn't be better provided within the work setting. They questioned whether the time and effort of a preservice program would provide the units with advantages we felt it would. Their questions were answered in February, 1966, when the program design was presented.

The next phase of development of the program was a meeting with the leadership teams to discuss what additions or modifications they saw as being essential to the program to prepare the staff for a particular unit.

THE PRESERVICE PROGRAM: HIGHLIGHTS AND ISSUES

The program philosophy, objectives for trainees, objectives for the trainers, teaching methods and the content and flow of the program may be found in Appendix A.

There are several areas I would like to highlight at this time. First, while many people participated in presenting seminars and other sessions, one chief trainer remained constant. (In all but one service, I did this.) This process seemed necessary so that the trainees had the feeling that there was one central person who was interested in them and their learning process. I also served as a role model for them in that I was able to stop a speaker for questioning, clarification, or disagreement. Second, the heaviest emphasis in the teaching method was on an experiential base for all learning. Thus, exercises such as role playing were frequently used to assess knowledge gained from reading and seminars and to provide the group with actual (rather than hypothetical) data on which to base discussion. Third, group dynamics training was considered the foundation not only of training for patient care but, even more important, for team formation. Both the Tavistock method and sensitivity training, with a focus on interpersonal competence, decision making, group formation, and cohesiveness, were used. [12,14] Sensitivity training was used as the consistent model after the first two sessions since it was found that the Tavistock method, focusing authority relationships and group dynamics from a more analytic point of view, was not as useful for staff groups as it has been for more sophisticated groups in leadership. Further evaluation of this decision is needed since a major issue for individuals and staff groups as a whole is their response to those in authority positions.

It is important to look at some of the issues that may result from the kind of training I have discussed. First, when all levels of personnel are trained together there is a period of time in the transition from training to service during which individuals and the group as a whole have difficulty allowing leadership that comes from within. For example, as teams are formed and a team leader (who might be a nurse or a psychiatric aide) is designated, both the designated leader and the remainder of the group have to test out the new relationships. Second, staff trained together in this manner are strongly cohesive, can support one another, and may find it difficult to rearrange their group boundaries to include members from other disciplines on the team. Third, while the leader may be impressed with the level of competence exhibited by the staff he may not be prepared to deal with the shared leadership the group may demand. All of these problems occurred in our setting and have taken varying lengths of time to be resolved. Another serious issue which emerges when staff have been trained together and when they are encouraged to work at their highest level of competency is that they continue to receive different levels of financial reward. That is, even if a nonprofessional becomes a team leader in the setting he still is likely to receive less pay than the professional for the responsibility he is assuming.

CURRENT PROGRAM

When the Center was opened an extensive and successful preservice program was provided. Since then, varying models have been attempted to maintain a preservice base as new employees have entered the system. These attempts have been fraught with many difficulties. First, employee turnover is erratic; thus some people might be in the system several months before a program is offered. Second, staff could no longer be trained to work together on any given unit since, in a group of fifteen new staff members, all units might be represented. Third, service demands made it impossible for any unit to keep a new employee on the day shift for three months while at the same time releasing him for the training program. After attempting several models of central training, the clinical specialists on the various units asked that they be allowed to try their own intraunit training for new employees. This has been done for the past year.

Continuing education has been continued since the staff have high expectations for continued learning, a feeling in part based on the investigative attitude stimulated and fostered through the earlier learning experiences. As the nursing role has expanded at the Center, there has also been demand for new learning so that learning experiences have been necessary for the director of nursing through to the staff level. Continuing education is primarily the responsibility of the clinical specialist on each unit, with the associate director serving as a resource person. No Center-wide education programs have been instituted without consultation and agreement from the clinical specialists. One such program conducted in the summer and early fall of 1969, used 16 films from Video Nursing, Inc.[15] These films were well received and many staff members have asked that selected films be shown again. Individual and group supervision is also used in continuing education with supervision from nurses or from members of other disciplines depending on the nature of the learning needed. Group supervision places people who have similar interests and skills together; thus medical students in clinical clerkship often participate in group dynamics supervision with nursing personnel, and social workers, nurses, and psychiatric aides may share family work supervision.

NEW CAREERS PROGRAM

One current program I would like to mention briefly is a new careers program. The trainees in this program all come from the inner city and are engaged in both an academic program through the local antipoverty agency and on-the-job training at the CMHC. The associate director for training is responsible for this program at the Center while the total directorship of the program rests in the antipoverty agency. The trainees are in the academic section of the program 16 hours each week and at the CMHC 24 hours. At the CMHC they are on specified units nineteen and one half hours and have three one and one-half hour classes. These classes have to do with: group dynamics training, social systems as they relate to mental health, and clinical conference. Classes were designed to augment their on-the-job training and also to provide generic training so that at the end of the program they might work in other agencies or in the community as well as at the Center itself.

The objectives of the New Careers Movement" are to (1) provide new skills and new jobs for the unemployed, (2) help alleviate the critical shortage of workers in human service areas, and (3) provide change in the way services are delivered. It is becoming apparent at the CMHC, as well as across the country, that these varying purposes may be in serious conflict with one another. The conflicts have been clearly identified by Kurzman who points out that, "as a new staff member, the paraprofessional is more likely to be absorbed into the structure than to become a successful advocate for change in the structure itself."[16] The same author further quotes Wilcox as follows: "Evidence points to the fact that these aides come into conflict with the employing agencies when they behave like 'legitimate locals,' the presumed reason for which they were hired. On the other hand, when they behave as staff members, the agency is more content, but the sub-professionals lose their presumed effectiveness."[17] Kurzman goes on to say ". . . potential for work simplification and the partial relief of our critical manpower problem may prove to be a strong asset. On the other hand, its potential for reducing the accountability of public agencies to their clients and for fostering an imbalance between social service and social action deserves thoughtful attention."[18]

Nursing leaders and others responsible for new careers programs will have to look at these questions seriously and decide on ways in which the conflicting purposes of the new careers movement may be managed.

SUMMER TRAINING PROGRAM FOR
INNER CITY YOUTH

The training program for inner city youth, conducted in the summer of 1969, might be seen as a type of "New Careers Training." Ten high school students from the inner city were employed in positions allocated by the state of Connecticut to the CMHC, and financed by Community Progress, Inc. The objectives of this program were: (1) To enable the students to earn money; (2) to increase the employment potential of the teenager; (3) to enable the students to learn new skills; (4) to introduce inner city youth to the mental health field; (5) to perform needed work for the CMHC; (6) to encourage a more positive self-image development; and (7) to broaden and deepen their career preparation.

The students in the program worked a 35-hour week as do other employees. During employment interviews they were given a wide range of job choices including positions as psychiatric aides, secretaries, public education and information aides, food service helpers, and assistants in plant operations. All except three chose the clinical area. Two of the three exceptions later transferred to clinical units and one left the program.

In addition to their job experience, all students had an individual supervisor and from their work placement area; all supervisors previously had volunteered to participate in the program. The group also met for one and one-half hours each week for a conference with the associate director of nursing and the assistant director of social work. Conference topics were chosen by the students after the first two sessions and ranged from questions about mental illness to discussions about how they would go about getting into college to prepare further in the mental health field. All the students who stayed in the program have maintained informal contact with the assistant director of social work or the associate director of nursing, and their academic motivation has increased. Those who are seniors in high school have been applying to colleges, something they say they had been discouraged from doing in the past.

SUMMARY

I have focused on the philosophy and objectives for any training program and some of the principles followed in the training program at the CMHC. The actual preservice program conducted at the CMHC is included as an appendix because I feel that if we study the process of program development and the foundation on which a program is built, the content and methods will flow from there.

I must stress at this time that those of us responsible for training in community mental health nursing carry a heavy responsibility for expanding the definition of psychiatric nursing practice; at the same time, we must be preparing people at all levels to fulfill the growing responsibilities in prevention, treatment, and rehabilitation. In designing programs, we should foster the individual's potential for contribution and not separate people in training on the basis of job classification. If we do not take this responsibility, the nonprofessional may be removed from the nursing services as has happened in some states. Furthermore, if we cannot broaden our scope on creative training and use of all levels of employees, we will find ourselves in the position of having less impact on the developing program in community mental health.

However, joint training of nursing personnel needs to be tested in other settings since, at the CMHC, many of the psychiatric aides were students or very creative community people. Some separate training through new careers training programs may be necessary to facilitate later joint training programs.

Growth in the training staff also is an important product of any training program. As the people responsible for training have continued experience, changes in philosophy are likely to occur which call for reassessment of parts of a program or the total program.

APPENDIX A

PRESERVICE PROGRAM–CONNECTICUT MENTAL HEALTH CENTER

Philosophy

1. All levels of nursing personnel have a valuable contribution to make to the treatment team and should not be limited in their activities and functions

except at the professional level, as required by law.

2. The potential of each individual should be maximized through training which is open on the basis of interest, capacity, and skills, and not on the basis of position.

3. At the present time we are simultaneously engaged in the processes of training, experimentation, and implementation, and this requires openness and flexibility in all aspects of program development.

4. Each individual, sick or well, has strengths and experiences that should be identified along with areas in which he needs assistance.

5. The agency in which individuals are employed must take responsibility for comprehensive training in order to prepare the employee to offer quality service.

Objectives for Trainees

A. The objectives of the program were established to assist the trainees in the following areas:

1. Orientation to the CMHC, including the establishment of a working agreement which clearly defines our expectations and delineates what we would offer in the program.

2. Reinforcement of positive attitudes and behavior and modification of those which were negative.

3. Delineation of the evolving philosophy and values of the CMHC.

4. Increased awareness of self as it related to working relationships—staff-patient, and staff-staff.

5. Awareness of group process, with a primary focus on small groups.

6. Creation of working units (team functioning).

7. Recognition of and ability to work with anxieties created when working with the mentally ill.

8. Recognition of the continuum of mental health and illness.

9. Conceptualization of, and appreciation for, the meaning of community mental health practices and services.

10. The development of ability to provide essential nursing care to meet the needs of the mentally ill individual.

11. The development of ability to formulate and execute nursing care plans.

Objectives for Trainers

In addition to content objectives the trainers' objectives were to assess the trainees according to the following criteria:

1. Entering behavior of the trainees as it related to training needs.

2. Competence in interpersonal relationships.

3. Attitudes, values, and beliefs of trainees.

4. Personality strengths and weaknesses (including maturity).

5. Special aptitudes and interests of trainees.
6. Complimentarity among members.

(Ultimately, the inservice program was to be based on assessments made in the preservice program and on a more definitive identification of task requirements as the program of each unit were established.)

Teaching Methods

1. Seminar presentations and discussion: presentations were provided by the trainers, outside leaders (senior nurses, psychiatrists, social workers, and community leaders), and the trainees themselves.
2. Films: these ranged from general films such as *Bold New Approach* to a film montage (which I compiled with Alberta Jacoby, executive director of the Mental Health Film Board) of specific interactions between a patient and professional or nonprofessional worker.
3. Role playing: this demonstrated both spontaneous and planned role playing. It included individual and group situations as well as staff-patient and staff-staff interactions.
4. Supervised clinical practice followed by clinical conferences.
5. Training in group dynamics, provided through a group experience for the entire training group.
6. Community exploration: this was provided by hearing about the community from agencies and leaders in the community and by the trainees visiting both office and nonofficial community agencies and resources.
7. Individual supervisory and evaluation conferences.
8. Weekly evaluations of the training program by the Trainees. (See Appendix B) These evaluations were used by the trainers to evaluate the effectiveness of the program. While alternations in the program were not always made when dissatisfaction was evident or when the trainees wanted more of a particular type of experience, the trainers were always careful to give feedback to the trainees about the weekly evaluations they had completed.

Content and Flow of the Program

The program was divided roughly into four phases:
PHASE 1: Orientation–2 weeks (80 hours)
1. Orientation to the Connecticut Mental Health Center
2. Growth and Development, primarily focusing on work of Erik Erikson and Selma Fraiberg (14 hours)
3. Interpersonal relationships as related to their experiences preceding the Connecticut Mental Health Center, and beginning concepts of interpersonal relationships in psychiatry. (12 hours)
4. Material relating to their specific units (i.e., concepts of day hospitalization,

24-hour care or crisis intervention). (A part of the 20-30 hours of orientation.)

PHASE 2: Clinical Practice—6 to 8 weeks (Approximately 90-116 hours)

1. Clinical site: A site for clinical training was chosen in which the program for the service could most nearly be approximated. Trainees spent three consecutive half days per week engaged in supervised clinical practice.

2. Clinical Conferences (approximately 30-40 hours): Supervisors of clinical practice conducted one and a half hour clinical conferences following each day of clinical practice. Focuses of the conference have been:
   a. What occurred that day.
   b. Relationship of their clinical practice to how they would function on their units.
   c. Relationship of their form of clinical practice to types of illnesses represented by the patients.

3. Illness Categoris (Approximately 30-40 hours): During the clinical practice phase, at least three hours per week have been devoted to a study of types of psychiatric illnesses. Trainees have been assigned specific readings, seminars have been presented by psychiatrists, followed by discussions of the meaning of the knowledge they have gained as applied to nursing care.

4. Family dynamics (approximately 15 hours): The social work staff assisted us in training for this area. We concentrated on the effects of family dynamics as they related particularly to family-patient interaction on the unit and the nurse's role in dealing with this area.

PHASE 3: Gaining knowledge of community Hospital Services—1 to 4 weeks (approximately 4½ to 20 hours) This area has been taught by having community leaders and resources (for example, director of the Visiting Nurse Association, executive chairman of the Community Council, police officers, chief nurses, state of Connecticut, Mental Health Association, and so on) speak to the groups, and also by having the trainees explore the Greater New Haven area, getting to know particular areas by visiting them in teams and driving or walking through the communities.

PHASE 4: Plans for Opening—(20-40 hours): For the most part the last two to three weeks of each program have been spent in discussion and physical planning for receiving patients. One of the teaching methods used during this period was role-playing the unit's program from the admission of the patient through planning for care.

Group Experience—(12-20 hours)

Each group of trainees was provided with a group experience, three of which were co-led by senior staff members at the Center who had a particular knowledge of group process plus one with a single trainer. The purposes for including such an experience were:

1. To learn about group dynamics through experience so that on those units

where nurses were participating in group care they would have a greater understanding of what was occurring in the patient groups.
2. To assist the staff in looking at how group dynamics affect working relationships in their units. For three of the services, this experience began in the second week of training and continued throughout; one unit began training the seventh week.

APPENDIX B

PRESERVICE TRAINING

You are now engaged in a training program designed to assist you in becoming a more competent and knowledgeable practitioner and team member. Every learning experience should be geared to the needs of the student when this is feasible. Therefore, evaluation and modification of the program becomes necessary in order to enhance its effectiveness.

We are using this device as one of our "feedback" mechanisms. We need your cooperation.

Please answer the following questions as succinctly and honestly as you can.

Thinking only of this week:

1. Which session or sessions were most helpful to you? Why?
2. Which experience or experiences were most difficult or upsetting to you?
3. What disappointments have you had to date?
4. Describe any significant reaction that you have had to the group?
5. What suggestions would you make for changes next week?

REFERENCES

1. Brown, A.F. Curriculum Development, 1st ed, Philadelphia, W.B. Saunders Company, 1960, Ch. 4.
2. Cotrell, C.J., Principles of Curriculum Construction, Aspects of Curriculum Development. Paper presented at 1961 Regional Meeting of Council of Member Agencies of the National League for Nursing, Department of Diploma and Associate Degree Programs. New York, National League for Nursing, 1962.
3. The Random House Dictionary of the English Language, College Edition, New York, Random House, Inc., 1968.
4. The American Heritage Dictionary of the English Language, 1st ed, Boston, Houghton Mifflin Company, 1969.
5. Brown, op. cit., p. 120.
6. Ibid.

7. Statement on Psychiatric Nursing Practice. Psychiatric Mental Health Nursing Division, New York, American Nurses' Association, 1967.
8. Ibid, p. 6.
9. Kennedy, J.F. Mental Illness and Mental Retardation, Message from the President of the United States, 1963.
10. Hollingshead, A. and Redlich, F. Social Class and Mental Illness, A Community Study, New York, John Wiley & Sons, Inc., 1958.
11. Klerman, G.L., Mental Health and the Urban Crisis. Amer. J. Orthopsychiat., 39:818-826, October, 1969.
12. Bion, W.R., Experiences in Groups, New York, Basic Books, Inc., 1961.
13. Rice, A.K. Learning for Leadership, Tavistock, 1965.
14. Bradford, L.P., Gibb, J.R., and Benne, K.D., eds. T-Group Theory and Laboratory Method. Innovation in Re-Education, New York, John Wiley & Sons, Inc., 1964.
15. Video Nursing, Inc. This project was supported by Improvement in Nursing Training, Grant No. NPG-114-04, Division of Nursing, USPHS, Department of Health, Education, and Welfare.
16. Kurzman, P., The New Careers Movement and Social Change. Social Casework, January 1970, 51:22-27.
17. Ibid. p. 25.
18. Ibid. p. 26.

DISCUSSION

Comment:

We are in the beginning stages of an inservice training program called "community caretakers." We take groups of people who have high impact on population—the clergy, for example—and we use many of the same methods mentioned, but they are not as refined or as well developed. I became aware, as you were talking, that you were training more people than we have on our staff. However, what is crucial for all community mental health workers to realize is that, somewhere and in some ways, we have to be much more conscious of the two-way street of training. I've learned a great deal from trainees in our program.

Comment:

I have also found this to be true. In fact, our particular mode of team training, operation, and treatment has been derived from the paraprofessional staff. Initially I would have said that it wouldn't work but it does work very effectively. I have observed a naturalness and spontaneity that we've long ago lost or that has been trained out of us.

Comment:

I suspect that one of the things that paraprofessionals are doing spontaneously is getting involved in social action. As nurses we must take a decision as to whether or not we too will be involved in social action. Problems arise when professionals become involved in social action because they are frequently representatives of official agencies.

Comment:

If social action is an appropriate means of involvement, then we need to help train people toward making the correct decisions relative to the actions they may take which affect the community. I can give you an example of what happens when you are involved. The community organization team of one of our local units helped a group of welfare mothers organize and subsequently they marched on the City Welfare Department. Some of our staff members were there and were arrested along with some of the mothers. The news of these events went up to the state welfare agency. Then the chief of the state welfare department challenged the Commissioner of Mental Health regarding one department fighting another. There was an attempt to terminate people from their duties. Finally, the director of nursing and the clinical director supported these people, saying, "They were doing what they were supposed to be doing and therefore this institution will support them." The incident has had continuing impact on us.

Question:

Have you had any experience with repercussions from community members and other agencies regarding your treatment methods, your kind of groups, questioning who you are, and whether you are qualified?

Comment:

We're just beginning to feel this and I think we're going to hear much more of this kind of thing. For example, there are many publications out for and against encounter groups and sensitivity training. Sensitivity training is a very touchy subject; we are being asked to change our vocabulary. Any kind of group which affects behavior and attitudes is very threatening and repercussions result.

Comment:

In the area of specialized training, staff nurses wanted to know more about psychopharmacology. We developed a staff program taught by a psychiatric staff member nationally known for his expertise in psychopharmacology. There was a specific nursing need not shared by other mental health workers, so separate sessions were necessary. All mental health workers need to have a fair amount of knowledge about medication even though they're not dispensing drugs. They must observe and understand the effects of the drug on the patient.

Comment:

I think we're talking about broader concepts. What does the nurse bring that is specific? Why don't we just educate community mental health workers? My own thinking is that the nurse brings with her a special background, as does any worker, and she also has a knowledge and experience which enables her to contribute and profit in a combined training program. We're not trying to make everybody a nurse, or a nurse a psychologist, or whatever—we're just enlarging common factors and I think the minute we get uptight and start protecting our field, we run into things like, "don't walk into my area, or past my boundaries." We have much to learn from one another.

Comment:

It really is a fallacy that once you put anybody in a training program he can stay where you want him. There are people called lay counselors from various communities, who have anywhere from eighth grade education through high school. You involve them in a certain kind of training depending upon where you want them to work. These people go through a typical crisis identity; they no longer speak the same language, they approach problems differently, in a sense, they are no longer in their community. They may be part of it but they don't have the same identity.

Comment:

I think we've moved into a period when we feel we're all equal but that it's a fallacy to say that we're all equal. I think it depends on who you are, where you are, and the time factor. I think right now we are experiencing condescending attitudes on the part of many professionals. It's not fair to the indigenous worker to say one thing and mean something else. It's all very well to have the philosophy which emphasizes that the indigenous worker *is* valuable. I don't think the indigenous worker even wants to be considered equal because he'd like that little piece of paper too, and wonders why they have developed the program the way they have. He often asks, "Why don't they make it possible for the indigenous worker to obtain his diploma or degree?" Many of them do want to go on and get an educational degree.

Comment:

I feel very strongly because we've just been through this kind of condescending, phony attitude at our particular center. The indigenous workers can really see through it. They have their own grapevine and they don't believe what one of our doctors said—that, "my degree is a handicap." People only say that if they have the degree, then there is no blurring of salaries. I'm fed up with the anti-intellectual, the anti-educational, prejudiced people who already have the education. It's like the middle-class people who down the middle-class values because they already have those things that are seen as highly important in this society. I thought about this when we heard earlier about "the lack of inhibition and the natural spontaneity." I think we also have to be very much attuned to the difficulty that the nonprofessional workers have. They may be working with a conflict and many problems; and keeping in mind their personal problems and employment trends, they need to have a counselor and a confidante, or they are labeled out of the system.

Mrs. French:

I want to comment on one of the things which has been a part of the "phoniness" that we tried to keep a handle on. When we say that we're not training people separately according to discipline, and so on, very often that sounds as though everyone is thrown into the same group regardless of where they are with their own knowledge and expertise. We have advanced supervisory groups for people who have been in the system for awhile, who very definitely develop some competencies. The clinical specialist is responsible for assessing whether or not an employee is ready for particular types of supervision. They cannot get into just any group on their own. They receive supervision in a group where people are at about the same level. When a psychiatric aide has been involved in emergency treatment and has had a lot of individual supervision, he may be considered ready for an advanced group. Not every psychiatric aide will be considered ready at the same time. Because of a realistic fear on my part that the nonprofessional would be maintained as a nonprofessional by the institution, we see to it that the very bright, capable aides are urged to go back for more education. We assist them to go back for more formal preparation.

Comment:

I think the thing that we ignore is that the deprived community is upwardly mobile in aspiration, in the sense that the people want to be adequately compensated for the services they perform. Now, if keeping them indigenous means tying them to an inadequate standard of living—substandard housing and archaic schools—then I'll agree that we're not helping them.

Comment:

We're going to use the people we have, in the best way, particularly those of us in the areas where there is a lack of qualified people. No matter what the background of the nurse is, she needs to have a grasp of the social system of the patient; she has to focus beyond the patient or group, and she has to be alert to the people and institutions that impinge on the client's system.

In terms of a theoretical background, she needs to have some knowledge of systems theory; then she will know that she may be an intruder into the client's system, that is, a nurse therapist working with a family is a new member; she's entering a semi-static system that has maintained some equilibrium and if she comes in as a change agent, she must expect resistance to change. There will be an immediate reaction either to incorporate the therapist into the system, or expel her, because she is trying to alter the ongoing process. And anybody going into a system, if they have information about what happens when a new person enters the system, they are at least better prepared intellectually to deal with the results.

Comment:

In order to learn about systems, we're trying something new right now with our students, "throwing" in together trainees from all the different disciplines and saying, "This is your team; now, it's up to you to pick your leader regardless of discipline." This is a way of learning about power struggles in social systems and it is more forceful than sitting in a classroom or looking at a scale.

Implications for Nursing in the Training of Paraprofessional Workers in the Community Mental Health Setting

HILDA RICHARDS, E.M., R.N.

"The price of hating other human beings is loving one's self less."[1] This statement, made by Eldridge Cleaver, kept running through my mind as I made abortive attempts to focus on the writing of this paper. During the approach and passing of a Christmas season which brought no peace, and while awaiting the birthday of a gentleman named Martin Luther King, who had a dream that echoed of love and was answered with violence, I speculated as to the futility of a conference on community mental health nursing. I examined my need to participate in the game-playing, the navel nursing, the irrelevancies, kept alive by the argument of role and role definitions. Such mole-picking might be a stimulating pastime on a cold winter's eve, if it did not result in the narrowing of the human soul and disparagement of one's fellowman. But the alternative, the withdrawal from those with difficulties in sharing, in allowing others to join the "haves," would be to become a "nonbeing."

My task is to discuss the training and utilization of paraprofessional workers, a topic that along with the chatter about the ghetto and the inner city, fills the void at cocktail parties. Although momentarily it is true that being against the paraprofessional and the "new careers" movement is like being for sin and against motherhood, the topic arouses strong ambivalent feelings among nursing groups, who seem destined for self-destruction in the misguided pursuit of the false god, "professionalism." To reduce anxiety, I will attempt to show the interrelatedness of professional and paraprofessional utilization and training.

The professional group defines its purpose for being through the amalgamation of societal need, the public's view of the profession's role, and the profession's view of itself. In community mental health, when we look at need (as defined by the people with whom I am concerned), the sensitive giver of service may well panic. Rainwater sees the health professions as having little to contribute to the resolution of the major social problems, which he considers to be poverty and racial oppression. This, at a time when the community mental health movement" . . . involves the effort to move out into the community and bring to bear the best of the insights and humanistic perspectives of psychiatric thought."[2]

The entrance of the paraprofessional worker to the constellation of care givers may be the essential catalyst for redefinition of client need and the development of a pragmatic service model. He may not lead us to psychological Nirvana, but neither have the present caretakers helped us partake of the fruits of paradise.

To launch out into a sterile description of the new careerist, complete with job description (some of which is published elsewhere), would be of little use to you.[3] Perhaps a perspective can be accomplished if I present an overview of the Harlem Rehabilitation Center, where I, with others, am making haste slowly. In this way, I can share with you "where I'm at" in my views of the New Careers movement.

OVERVIEW OF THE CENTER

The group I have strong concern for is black; many of them are poor; all suffer from the ills caused by an imposed, devalued, social position. I agree with Carmichael, who says, "We are aware that it has become commonplace to pinpoint and describe the ills of our urban ghettos."[4] The social, political, and economic problems are so acute that even a casual observer cannot fail to see that something is wrong. While descriptions are plentiful, however, there remains a blatant timidity about what to do to solve the problems.

"Neither rain nor endless definitive costly reports nor stop-gap measures will even approach a solution to the explosive situation in the Nation's ghettos. This country cannot begin to solve the problems of the ghettos as long as it continues to hang on to outmoded structures and institutions."[5] The health system looms as a Goliath among these institutions.

No matter how health is defined, health needs are agreed by all to be the greatest among those who can least afford the services. In the cycle of poverty—second-class citizenship, social malfunctions, feelings of powerlessness, needs for multiple social and health services—it is often difficult to decide where the thrust for breakthrough should be made. Some feel, and I share their view, that if we are to be at all effective, massive energy must be expended over the entire circumference. In the six years that I have been part of the growth and development of the Harlem Rehabilitation Center, I have worked to concretize its philosophy and have attempted to conceptualize nursing participation in such a reality.

The Harlem Rehabilitation Center is a community-based facility, a Division of the Department of Psychiatry, Harlem Hospital Center. Its socio-psychiatric orientation attempts to integrate intraphysic, interpersonal, and social aspects of the person in a multiple-service framework. Its service goals are:

1. To develop and utilize socio-psychiatric group rehabilitation approaches to provide social, psychiatric, educational, vocational, and community services to persons discharged from psychiatric hospitals and/or with severe chronic mental illness.
2. To provide related rehabilitation services and assistance to family and community individuals and groups in order to assist, directly or indirectly, in the rehabilitative process.
3. To serve as a force for individual, group and social change through the operation of preventive, habilitative and rehabilitative systems and their transactions with other social systems, directed toward altering psychological and/or social disorder.
4. To develop and implement relevant and effective systems of human service, participating in the development with other members of the professional, paraprofessional, and lay communities including recipients of service.[6]

These goals are incorporated in two service programs: The Psychiatric Program and the Vocational Rehabilitation Program; a Research and Evaluation Program and a Training and Education Program. Multiple approaches are central to service; thus, social, community, medical and psychiatric services are provided automatically.

Far beyond this (and as important as helping clients build occupational skills), our goals are to assist clients in building skills in: (1) developing and using new concepts and new cognitive systems; (2) assimilating new data about oneself and the world, so that these are connected to old data; (3) testing perceptions and mediations through acting with newly acquired behavior; and (4) managing varying degrees of stresses.

Intrinsic to rehabilitative approaches is the systems model where group involvement is necessary. Although it is not the primary aim of therapeutic and educational groups to promote social action, such group approaches in deprived communities can move a person from unproductive individual isolation to more successful action with and through the group.

In every aspect of our service, the "Paraprofessional Rehabilitation Worker" is the basic therapeutic staff member. Indeed, our hope is that, through the identification process, client behavior will be accelerated, that the longing to resemble will blossom, for we feel that, "The word which we shall make our own is the word whose echo we have heard within ourselves."[7]

If we backtrack for a moment and re-examine the agency's service goals we will see their relationship to some of the services that Schwartz and Schwartz have discussed under outpatient and ex-patient systems.[8] For purposes of analysis, I have presented a few of the service offerings in schematic form (see Tables 1, 2 and 3). These are: resocialization, sociotherapeutic approaches, and vocational rehabilitation (these are seen to form a continuum of rehabilitation); crisis intervention, short-term approaches, consultation, and community organization. I have listed what I see as essential ingredients of each system of service: goals of service; nature of clients served; physical location of service; intervention assessment; examples of activities involved; process used by helping person; and, some of the skills and knowledges needed to perform activity.

I have presented them in this manner so that, at a glance, one can see that the service model being developed at our Center has broad application for community mental health and for nursing. Through a minute dissection of the systems ingredients listed, one can begin to envision the types of skills needed by persons involved as service agents, and the knowledge and skill which must be part of their formal education, or which must be given as part of their training.

A few years ago I stated that nurses, as a result of some 20 years of experience with paraprofessional workers in the hospital setting, had something to bring to the training of Psychiatric Rehabilitation Workers. Nurses had something to bring these workers because of their ability to transmit knowledge in a meaningful manner through guidance, conferencing, and "on-the-spot" teaching.[9] My beliefs seem reinforced when I examine nursing and paraprofessional functioning in our setting. Here, the psychiatric nurse becomes involved in and often spearheads a variety of therapeutic approaches. Along with the Psychiatric Rehabilitation Worker, she participates in: family therapy, home visiting, crisis intervention, and health education; the interpretation of the social system to the client, the family, and other professionals; community organization and community action; consultation to agencies, and professional and lay groups. One of the prime assets the nurse brings to this setting and to the training of others is her willingness and ability to learn and participate in activities not traditionally considered part of the nursing role. That seems ironic, at a time when specialization and narrowing of role definition are hailed as virtues!

While it is evident that nurses bring much to the training of the paraprofessional group, I have altered my previous position somewhat. I no longer see these workers as merely an essential link to bridging the gap between middle-class therapist and lower income patients. I am now more aware of their potential as a developing group who can broaden services in the mental health field by means of their ability to tap strengths of clients and community.

The concept of New Careers carries little meaning unless it allows for both vertical and horizontal movement. Still another choice component included

Table 1.

EXAMPLES OF PSYCHIATRIC-MENTAL HEALTH SERVICES OFFERED AT THE HARLEM REHABILITATION CENTER
(with application to other settings)

System Ingredients	Resocialization	Socio-Therapeutic	Vocational
Goals	To increase levels of social functioning, improve coping behavior, communication skills; reappraise reality	Same; with more stress on skills learning necessary in everyday life	To improve work capacity
Nature of Clients	Appropriate to all patients and clients, depending on specific needs and level of functioning		
Location of Service	Day Care Center Rehabilitation Center	Day Care Center Rehabilitation Center	Vocational Rehabilitation Center; psychiatric Rehabilitation Center; Sheltered Workshop.
Intervention Assessment	Improve problem-solving capacity in Center; at home; in community	Same, plus improve skill knowledge and evaluate stress level	To increase stress capacity to allow for working; to teach skill knowledge

Activities	Group meetings; group projects; planned and executed recreational activities; implementation of therapeutic community concept; home visiting; community meetings; organizing actions	Same, plus remedial skills; organized adjustment activities; activities exploring creativity	Pre-vocational evaluation and training; vocational training and job placement; group and individual counseling; therapeutic community meetings; social, psychiatric and health services
Process Used	Crisis intervention, advocacy roles; group methods; community organization	Same, plus teaching	Teaching, evaluation; interpersonal counseling; group therapy
Skills and Knowledge	1. Group therapy—process 2. Learning theories 3. Assessment of strengths and dysfunctioning areas of individual and family 4. Physical-emotional health 5. Crisis intervention 6. Deviancy-health illness continuum	Same, plus specific knowledge, (tutoring sewing, crafts)	1. Vocational knowledge about evaluation and skill training 2. Knowledge of stress points in training 3. Crisis—psychological reactions 4. Physical-emotional health 5. Learning theories

Table 2.

EXAMPLES OF PSYCHIATRIC-MENTAL HEALTH SERVICES
OFFERED AT THE HARLEM REHABILITATION CENTER
(with application to other settings)

System Ingredients	Crisis	Short-Term Approaches
Goals	To help person or family regain equilibrium at same or higher level of integration	To increase levels of social functioning; reappraise reality.
Nature of Clients	All types; more often used with lower and middle income clients	Those with situation reactions to personal or social situations; neurotics
Location of Service	Store front; emergency room service; suicide prevention centers; home visiting crisis	Clinic or home
Intervention Assessment	Diagnose difficulty; handle problem on sport; decide what kind of help is needed in the future; establish person in facility or with helping person	To increase communications help individual or family redefine problem; focus on strength
Activities	Interview—individual or group	Short-term, individual or group therapy; vestibule groups; short-term family therapy; family treatment in home
Process Used	Interpersonal, interactional— at appropriate stage of crisis	Interpersonal transactional group; repressive-supportive constructive approach; self-development
Skills and Knowledges	1. Stages of crisis 2. Responses to crisis 3. Knowledge of intervention methods	1. Focal point of therapeutic operation 2. Role and function of leader 3. Stages of group and related themes being dealth with 4. Ability to do assessment of individual and family strength and areas of dysfunctioning

should be: at a certain point, the worker should be able to either move into an established profession or remain to assist in professionalizing his own group. We have attempted to develop paraprofessional sub-roles to allow for both these aspects. The various sub-roles are: Health Service Worker, Socio-therapeutic Activities Worker, Case Service Worker, Community Worker, and Vocational Worker. Among the processes used (and I refer you again to Tables 1, 2, and 3), are intervention, advocacy, community involvement, teaching, counseling, group leading, evaluation, support, and education. The behavior of paraprofessionals with clients reveals commitment; and incorporates those elements

Table 3.

EXAMPLES OF PSYCHIATRIC-MENTAL HEALTH SERVICES
OFFERED AT THE HARLEM REHABILITATION CENTER
(with application to other settings)

System Ingredients	Consultation	Community Organization
Goals	To help clients identify and resolve own conflicts	To help clients tap their own strengths; improve coping behavior
Nature of Clients	Any group of caretakers–clergy, police; may include supervisor-supervisee relationship	Any group of community people having common problem, this includes persons called patients
Location of Service	Any place, any agency, including schools; general hospital	In community, block, school, apartment building, and so on; organization in community
Intervention Assessment	To help caretakers improve functioning; to help build in help for psycho-social problems in non-treatment institutions	To help persons identify and organize around workable, commonly-held problems
Activities	Short-term workshops teaching agency assessment; field visits; staff or patient-staff assessment	Organizing block, tenement, building; PTA members
Process Used	Consultation and education	1. Organizing and agitating 2. Adversary and redress 3. Program development
Skills and Knowledges	1. Focal point of intervention; guide clarify and extend perceptions 2. Role of leader 3. Stages of group and themes 4. Change theory	1. Principles and practices of community organization 2. Principles of preventive psychiatry

essential to a positive relationship: respect, involvement, and the empathy of the helping person for the client.[10]

Let me support this point with two quotes from papers written by paraprofessional workers. An Activity Worker, writing about her pride in being able to teach sewing, writes: "I feel that this is a great therapeutic value to people who are mentally ill. Many people are judged by their clothing, especially in a poor ghetto area. Not knowing the value of a wellmade garment, many people shop for quantity, since they do not know the value of quality. When I show them how to cut out the front and back of a dress, they can remember this, because they have some sense of self-pride, and beauty. Remember, we are living in an economically poor neighborhood, where most of the time, a welfare recipient cannot afford a dress. It gives them a chance to feel that they are part of society, to be able to put on a new dress that was not bought from a Harlem Thrift Shop. My greatest desire is to be able to help myself, and to help others to be able to face many of the problems that occur daily."[11]

In her paper, a Health Service Worker recounts her difficulties in obtaining adequate medical care for clients, and discusses some of her experiences in home visiting. She concludes with these statements: "This is the most thrilling position I have held in my whole life. It is as exciting as seeing a child walk, or hearing him talk for the first time. You become so involved with the patients that you see them as close friends. Above all, you are helping a human being to find himself, so that he can enjoy some of the beautiful things our world has to offer."[12]

On an operational level, commitment includes a person's uniqueness and intrapsychic dynamics, his view of the world and the people in it, and the interrelations among various aspects of his external world. At the Center, we have incorporated these elements in our criteria for screening applicants: concern for the black community, awareness of the problems of ghetto living, relatedness of life experience, and ability to function in a constructive manner. Life experience is seen as more important than formal education. Indeed, the trainee can have no education beyond high school, nor is the diploma necessary for entrance level positions.

Some would like to think that commitment alone is responsible for our low turnover. But commitment, like love, is not enough. For many, this is the first time that they have had a job which combines respect for the person and respect for his background of experience—where the fact that he has a prison record, is an ex-alcoholic, or has been on welfare is an asset, rather than a liability. Of course, he is also given the normal American incentive of a decent salary and the possibility for advancement.

At present, there are four grades in the Career Ladder: Trainee, Worker, Technician and Specialist. Each position has its specific requirements, and these are written in a way that does not box a person in with tight educational requirements.

The first three months of employment is considered the orientation period. During this time, on-the-job training is combined with sessions using (as much as possible) the interactional, small group workshop method. Core training includes some areas familiar to nurses and others in which more familiarity would be a decided asset.

A sampling of topical areas in the core training are: growth and development; the black family in America; concepts of anxiety and mental health; crisis and crisis intervention; the process of rehabilitation; the black experience; basic body systems and functioning; alcoholism and addiction. Workshops are held in the areas of group process and group participation, therapeutic community, the principle and practices of socio-psychiatric rehabilitation, and the dynamics of individual, group, and organizational change.

The workshops continue throughout employment and are combined with other aspects of inservice training, for example: techniques of rehabilitative services in specialized areas; self-development as a Rehabilitation Worker (sensitivity training, peer group conferences, remedial skills and self-development); individual and group supervision; supportive services.[13]

While it may be useful to discuss how we professionals train others, it might be even more valuable for us to look at training modifications brought about by lessons we have learned from workers.

The paraprofessional worker made us practice one of the truths we espoused—that one of the necessary behaviors needed for effective participation in our social system is to have control over one's own destiny so that planning is worthwhile. This is denied the consumer, as long as he is not included as a participant. Indeed, without it in the black community, the best services become paternalism, constantly fostering the centuries old, parent-child, black-white relationships.

The confrontations that developed led us to redefine therapeutic community implementations as a sharing of power in the Center itself. This is leading to planned structural modification, and such modification is necessary to meet the demands for real decision-making for client and worker, and for the incorporation of the New Careers.

A new service model also dictates institutional change. Advocacy seems to be central to the concept which synthesizes both the conflict and accommodative modes. An advocate, according to Webster, is one who supports and pleads for another. In fact, the worker often assists the client as he negotiates for services that are his right. The process uses rehabilitation and social action approaches.[14] The development of our service model has resulted from a merging of professional-paraprofessional orientation. It has affected content and method of training.

The professionals have learned their lessons well and, for the most part, have risen to the challenge of change. Personal involvement creates havoc with objective analysis. Yet it would not be inappropriate to say that what we have learned has modified the professional role; it has broadened our spectrum of awareness concerning true rehabilitation and the social restraints which block progress; and it has provided more adequate definitions of the mental health problems.

There is struggle, but the struggle is not without benefits. "The desire to participate on all levels as persons providing service—professional and paraprofessional, administrative and service, managerial and fiscal, technical and executive—could ultimately contribute to the resolution of a manpower shortage in human service, as well as to a change in the seat and structure of power. The manpower change alone will require, and ultimately bring about, modifications in the accrediting criteria, in access to technical and professional institutions, in acceptance of the educational value of life experiences, and in health and educational systems themselves—in short, in institutional change.[15] The development of a training program involves difficulties, but the difficulties cannot be compared to the obstacles that are involved in institutionalizing new roles.

We are presently working through the problems involved in having new job titles accepted by the New York City structure, the university, and the unions. Our greatest success has been with the university and with one of the unions since, structurally, they have more flexibility. Permanency necessitates Civil Service acceptance and our biggest thrust now is in that area.

Efforts have been made to relate our training program to a junior college system. Our investigations have reinforced our view that we are further ahead in our ideas and teaching approaches than are the traditional systems available to us. Thus, an idea like giving college credit for relevant life experience (which seems old to us), appears to be a radical idea in the educational framework.

IMPLICATIONS

Development of New Career training programs requires parallel changes in the role definitions of professionals and paraprofessionals, and a revision in professional education. Training for these workers can no longer be viewed as simply the induction of unskilled persons to do menial, dead-end jobs. Rather, training must allow for self-improvement activities—remedial skills and instruction for high school equivalency examinations, and personal counseling for workers needing supportive services. Sensitivity training has proved helpful for both professional and paraprofessional workers, for sharing and working through their anxieties and conflicts concerning roles, power, status, and their effectiveness in a shifting environment.

We say the professional is generally the supervisor; but what does it do to one's image as a supervisor when the person supervised is performing functions the professional himself would have difficulty with? It is not always easy, even in traditional settings, to see your student go beyond you.

Teaching others for roles for which we, ourselves, have not been prepared, is only one of many concerns. As the professional's vista broadens, he will see need for more knowledge of community organization, change theory, administration, the politics of interrelated institutional structures, the manipulations of budget, people, and systems, and the struggles underlying community control and urban problems. Clinicians traditionally have viewed these matters as beneath them; yet, these matters seem to be crucial to the existence (if not the success) of service. Are we as professionals, able to make the necessary role shifts? What does it mean in terms of our educational preparation? How do we keep a sense of sanity and a center of gravity amidst ambiguity and change? Are we able to teach for this?

I have tried to share a few of my ideas with you, my experiences and quandaries. I believe that the development of a relevant service model, particularly in the black community, necessitates the inclusion of the paraprofessional Psychiatric Rehabilitation Worker. Such a modification in the approach to service necessitates the re-examination of the perceptions and the value systems of the professional helping person. This confrontation may help professionals in their struggle to "love one another." According to Albert Camus, happiness is seen as the struggle toward the heights.[16] If, indeed, happiness is a struggle then we are all in bliss!

REFERENCES

1. Cleaver, E. Soul on Ice. New York, McGraw-Hill Book Company, 1968, p. 17.
2. Rainwater, L. Mental Health and Social Action. Presented at Dedication Ceremony of the Department of Psychiatry, Mental Health Center Division of the University of Rochester, Rochester, New York, September, 1969.
3. Christmas, J.J., Edwards, J., and Wallace, H. New Careers and New Mental Health Services: Fantasy or Future? Presented at American Psychiatric Association Conference. Miami, Florida, March, 1969.
4. Carmichael, S., and Hamilton, C.V. Black Power: The Politics of Liberation in America. New York, Vintage Books, 1967, p. 164.
5. Ibid.
6. Christmas, J.J. Socio-psychiatric Rehabilitation in a Black Urban Ghetto: Conflicts, Issues and Directions. Amer. J. Orthopsychiat., 39:651-661, July, 1969.
7. Bergson, H. The Two Sources of Morality and Religion. As quoted by Friedman, M.S. in To Deny Our Nothingness; Contemporary Images of Man, New York, The Delacorte Press, 1967, p. 363.
8. Schwartz, M.S., and Schwartz, C.G. Social Approaches to Mental Patient Care. New York, Columbia University Press, 1964.
9. Richards, H. The Role of the Nurse in the Therapy of the Lower Socioeconomic Psychiatric Patient. Perspect. Psychiat. Care, 5 (2) 82-91, 1967.
10. Gould, G.T. Toward a Philosophy of Personalized Care. In Interpersonal Relations, Maloney, E.M., ed., Dubuque, Iowa, William C. Brown Company, Publishers, 1966, pp. 12-13.
11. Stroy, R.M. A Bridge to Reality. Presented at the Remotivation Workshop, Essex County Overbrook Hospital, Cedar Grove, New Jersey, September, 1968.
12. Carter, H. The Role of the Health Service Worker. Presented at Institute on Voice of the Community at Columbia University School of Public Health and Administrative Medicine, January, 1969.
13. Christmas, J.J., Edwards, J. and Wallace, H. op. cit., p. 4.
14. Daniels, E., Social Rehabilitation as a Function of Community Action Programs. Prepared for presentation at the New York State District Conference of American Psychiatric Association, 1967.
15. Christmas, J.J. Obligations to High Priority Target Groups: Philosophical Implications. April 30, 1968.

16. Camus, A. The Myth of Sisyphus and Other Essays. New York, Vintage
     Books, 1959, p. 91.

ADDITIONAL REFERENCES

Richards, H. The Relationship between Group Approaches and Social Action
in Community Mental Health Settings. In Current Concepts in Clinical
Nursing, Vol. 2. St. Louis, Mo., The C.V. Mosby Co., 1969, p. 153-159.

Richards, H., and Daniels, M.S. Rehabilitation in the Black Ghetto: Innovative
Treatment Roles and Approaches. Amer. J. Orthopsychiat., 39 (4) July, 1969,
pp. 662-676.

DISCUSSION

Question:
  We have a great many black paraprofessionals in our system, and have had
many problems. It seems that our white, middle-class professionals selected the
bright, articulate, middle-class type from the ghetto communities. They might be
described as opportunists without real involvement in the community. We've
learned some lessons, but we still make mistakes in screening. I'm wondering
how white, middle-class professionals can avoid hiring paraprofessionals who are
not sincere about helping members of the community. Who screens and hires
your paraprofessionals?

Mrs. Richards:
  We have a review board which screens all applicants in groups. In this
group-screening process an attempt is made to select people we think will fit into
the setting. We select those people who are outgoing, have a commitment and
are able to wrestle with being black, being poor, being in, being out, and who are
not afraid of mental illness.
  One of the things that I have found over and over is that we professionals
tend to screen out rather than in. Once we hire a person, we try to build in the
kind of things that they need in order to function. Many applicants who want to
work as paraprofessionals at our hospital do not have a uniform or a pair of
shoes. The nursing staff have often brought in their own uniforms and obtained
a pair of shoes from the volunteer service to enable a paraprofessional to begin
work. Another example is an ex-addict on our staff who is wrestling about going
back on drugs. We talked with his parole officer and we are working to give him
the support he needs. Remembering that this is the first time he has ever had a
job that gave him dignity and selfworth and a decent income, we build in some
helping mechanisms rather than saying, "This is your problem, don't bring your
problems to work." We realize that most people do bring their problems to
work.

Question:

I have really been encouraged by your presentation. You are working in teams with the hardcore, unemployed black groups. I am wondering if your success is because your professionals are black and the paraprofessionals can identify with you?

Mrs. Richards:

That's part of it, although the worse people are white-black people, black people whose attitude and thinking are more white than black. We have some white staff who are just as involved. They are involved in a different way and for different reasons. We all have our own reasons for being there, but I think it is because the professionals are involved and share a common philosophy, whatever their color.

Question:

The utilization of the paraprofessional worker seems to have a two-fold purpose: one is to elevate the life-style of that particular person, and the other is the recognition that this person can communicate better with people he has lived with and shared similar experiences. I wonder, in your agency, if a particular paraprofessional has taken on the value system of the more educated person and starts to "move away from," does he then jeopardize the quality of his contributions?

Mrs. Richards:

This is a question that I am asked frequently. We have not found this to be true. In most systems, the paraprofessional is a sub-professional and therefore the value is to become a professional; that is, you do your thing, you earn our money, you move up, and therefore you must become one of us. In our system, we are both moving. Most of our professionals have not lost sight of the poor background we came from, we are changing our perceptions together. In addition, in our system you don't have to be a professional to earn a high income. Right now we are wrestling with the fact that some of our paraprofessionals earn more than some of our professionals. In a small system of 70 people, this is a struggle. In our system, the top man on the totem pole is the paraprofessional. We are involved in career training and change. The whole value system, the whole organizational structure is different from the usual.

Question:

We have a whole cadre of experienced people who have worked for 15 years with people identified as "mentally ill." They are in a position of having fewer opportunities in the New Careers program and they are bitter. What makes them so angry is that if they were ex-addicts they could earn $2,000 a year more as rehabilitation or drug counselors than they do for being "clean" for 15 years. Do you only hire the hardcore, unemployed who have been on welfare, and those with criminal records?

Mrs. Richards:

You're in trouble if you set up a system which excludes so many. In our system you do not have to be on welfare—but you can be. We have many nice, ordinary people. I mention the other types because many places report that black men are difficult to find to employ. We have had more success with men who have had records than with men who have not had records. The former have at least fought and struggled but have not been overcome by the system. Many who have not been overcome by alcohol or drugs (which keeps them non-functioning) have had to do the "fight-flight" bit.

Question:

You described a comprehensive training program for paraprofessional workers. Could you be more specific regarding what nursing has to offer your particular kind of rehabilitation workers, both in training and practice?

Mrs. Richards:

Some of this is in the paper and the schedules. I developed most of the content and philosophy of the training program, the whole orientation of observing behavior and focusing on experience which is nursing; this is in contrast to diagnostic entities; that is medicine and not generally useful. The concept of the health-illness continuum and concomitant services, assessment of strengths rather than weaknesses, and crisis theory and crisis intervention are all part and parcel of nursing. Our background in public health nursing, home visiting, and medical-surgical nursing is invaluable. It is not an "either-or" but an integrated knowledge of physical, psychological, and sociological phenomena.

Nurses are primarily attached to the health-service group. One of our roles, then, is to train people to assume the advocacy role related to getting health services, insuring that people get good physical health services. By the time you define health services broadly, the term covers a great many things; the health service worker primarily relates to major crisis situations. When others are frightened by the client, the nurse is called in to deal with the crisis. It's a whole system whose clients' lives revolve and evolve around crisis, requiring nursing to work through the dependency-independency conflict. These activities are carried out in the home setting and in the center. We are always helping workers observe, analyze, and assess behavior. I believe that, of all the professional groups, nursing has the most knowledge and skill which can be translated into action in working with people in low-income populations. We have the positive image; we have valuable knowledge and skills; why do we want to give this away to do other things? We put a premium on the "50-minute hour" (which isn't useful) to prove we are as good as the doctor—rather then providing the client with the care he needs.

Comment:

Because of our location, we do not have the power to recruit nurses that have a master's degree except for the administrative positions. We have many nurses on our staff who are hospital school, diploma graduates, and some who are baccalaureate graduates. What we do is write in the job description "baccalaureate degree, or the equivalent." We discussed what we mean by "the equivalent", since it can be interpreted either very loosely or very rigidly. We try to get across that the nurse needs to have a background in the social sciences. We try to incorporate the missing ingredients in our inservice education programs.

Comment:

We do not look at the nurses' level of education—we look at their personal qualifications; whether or not they can relate to people, and whether or not they've been successful with their own lives; whether or not they're flexible enough to get into a program are prepared to use their skills in collaboration with other people on the staff. We are interested in whether or not they are bright and willing to learn. We learn together here because things are happening too fast for us to go and get the necessary education elsewhere. We learn by reading the current literature. We bring in people who know about systems and change, and how these forces affect the various segments of the population we serve.

There is no question that the dynamic, bright, creative person ought to go on to school. The question is—are we giving the dynamic bright, creative person who is *not* going to go to school opportunities for growth?

Differential Role Development For Nurses in Group Therapy

JANELLE SMITH RAMSBURG, R.N., M.S.W.

A question frequently asked of and by nurses is, "Is there a place for the nurse as a group psychotherapist in an interdisciplinary setting?" At Western Missouri Mental Health Center the answer is a resounding "Yes!" Having reached this conclusion, the development of nurses who could function as group psychotherapists became an item of importance not only to the department of nursing but to the agency as a whole. Although this paper will be focused on the development program of one center, an attempt will be made to conceptualize the experience and arrive at generalizations which may be useful in a variety of settings.

The patient population of the Western Missouri Mental Health Center, located in the inter-city area of Kansas City, Missouri, is drawn from the lower half of the socioeconomic level of the city. As a comprehensive, community-oriented mental health center, Western Missouri offers a complete array of services. Group process is a major mode of treatment throughout the Center. While the need should not be minimized for nurses working in all areas of the center to understand and use group dynamics, this paper will describe the development of nurses as group psychotherapists in the outpatient department. Therefore, remarks about the organization and services of the center will be confined to a discussion of the group psychotherapy program in that department.

The program stresses rapid evaluation and treatment, and patients are assigned to treatment groups from any and all services. Assignment to groups is made largely on the basis of overt behavior and the products of that behavior and not on the basis of psychodynamic criteria or formal diagnostic classification. In keeping with the community-oriented focus of the Center, the aim of group treatment in the outpatient department is to increase effective social functioning.

Group therapists are drawn from the four major disciplines—medicine, nursing, social work, and psychology—in all clinical services. This serves to increase staff investment since patients are frequently referred to outpatient therapy by the same people who have been responsible for their inpatient service care or who will be responsible for their care if referral to another service becomes necessary.

A co-therapy approach is used in all group therapy situations in order to provide more adequate observation and therapeutic coverage. Additionally, this approach offers not only an excellent but a necessary training ground for prospective group psychotherapists. In assigning therapists, an attempt is made to obtain both a male and female therapist for each group and to select them from different disciplines.

All prospective therapists are expected to attend a basic program although training as a group therapist is considered a continuing process. The purpose of the basic program is to provide a setting in which the general concepts and fundamental skills of group therapy can be learned and applied, regardless of the therapist's theoretical frame of reference. Educational objectives for the program are thought of in terms of acquisition, application, analysis, synthesis, and evaluation of knowledge, as well as in terms of changes in interests, attitudes, values, and behavioral adjustments.

THE TRAINING PROGRAM

The four major clusters of activity in the training program include: a didactic seminar, a small group process experience, a supervised experience as a group psychotherapist, and a clinical workshop which takes the form of a demonstration group. The training program is interdisciplinary in nature; thus, participants are selected by disciplines. Currently all nurses attend the first two phases of the program. The experiences and information obtained in the first two seminars are considered useful in helping the nurse develop her capabilities more fully. Specifically, the seminars are considered useful to nurses working with patients in other than formal group psychotherapy situations. Those nurses selected to continue the remaining phases of the central program in group therapy include nurses responsible for planning patient care across service areas, nurses with advanced preparation, and nurses who have demonstrated special interest or talent in working with groups of patients. Frequently at the Center, nurses will be observed attempting to use group process in working with patients even though they may be unaware of the theoretical constructs underlying their efforts.

Group Process Seminar

While Mullan and others have indicated that personal group psychotherapy is a necessary experience in becoming a group psychotherapist, we believe that, unless there is a need for personal therapy, a small group experience in a group process seminar is sufficient.[1] The group process seminar focuses on feelings, perceptions, and reactions in the "here and now;" it does not encourage speculations about motivations or relationships outside of the group. Nurses who feel the need for personal psychotherapy are encouraged not to attend the seminar, but if a nurse is involved in personal therapy she is eligible for the group—provided her therapist agrees to her participation.

There are approximately twelve participants in each of the seminar groups. Each group meets with their co-leaders for a total of 40 hours. The groups meet weekly for 10 two and one half hour sessions. The additional 16 hours is consumed in two eight hour sessions, one at the beginning and one at the mid point of the seminar. While discussion continues as to whether this method is therapy or education in this setting, it is meant to provide an opportunity for both cognitive (intellectual) and affective (emotional) learning.

Even though the emphasis is on affective learning, opportunities for cognitive learning are not neglected. In a group process seminar, the distinctions between these two levels of functioning are necessarily clarified. The nurse participant begins to learn to consider the difference between the two processes in a manner that can be understood without being threatening to other members of the group. In addition, she has an opportunity to investigate her modes of interaction and her impact on group members, plus an opportunity to discover how it feels to be a group member and experience the various phases of the group's development. Briefly, the nurse participating in this phase of the program has an excellent opportunity to improve her group membership, leadership, and interpersonal skills.

Nurses may have particular difficulty with the affective learning experiences of the group process seminar. Generally, the nurse's previous educational preparation has taught her to empathic and understanding of other people but she seldom gives herself the same consideration. Further, if she has been fortunate enough to be in a program that did help her learn to identify her feelings, she frequently has been encouraged to suppress or cover these feelings rather than to express and examine them. Nurses, perhaps more than members of other disciplines, derive emotional support from their particular subgroup. Although the nursing subgroup is not available in this situation, the nurse will generally attempt to attach herself to another strong subgroup and let it carry her through the experience. She will not allow herself to get anything from the group, however, because she will not let them know what she is thinking or feeling. She may express her inability to cope with this aspect of the seminar by engaging in small talk, absenting herself from the group with varying pretexts, or by open rebellion. Rebellion among the nurses at the Center has ranged from verbal assaults on the total experience to sitting in a seething silence.

One unusual aspect of the experience offered at the Center is that the group may be made up of people who work together on various teams or who are otherwise clinically associated with each other. With the emphasis on the here and now, participants are likely to work out difficulties in relationships with people they will continue to see; the nurse may find this aspect of the seminar particularly threatening, few nurses have had previous experience in group situations. She may find herself in conflict between taking time out to improve the quality of her performance and meeting what she perceives as immediate and pressing service needs. She demonstrates the conflict by arriving late at each session with the explanation, "Something came up," apparently assuming that other members of the group will understand. She is frequently surprised, then hurt, then angry to find that, in fact, they do not understand. As I pointed out above, nurses at the Center have expressed their feelings of discomfort by vocally attacking individual members of the group, withdrawing behind a blank or bored facial expression, or leaving the group entirely.

Participants in general and nurses in particular may approach the small group experience with some anxiety. A dilemma for nursing education is how to encourage and support the nurse during this kind of experience while, at the same time, allowing her to gain maximum benefit from the group. Nurses have strong, informal communication links. Information coming through these channels is not always either accurate or supportive.

Recently, a nurse received a memorandum confirming her participation in the seminar and instructing her as to time, place and mode of dress. She turned to a nurse standing nearby and asked, "What do they mean by casual dress?" The second nurse replied, "They mean slacks. You"ll love it. You get down on the floor, roll around, and feel each other!" Part of the job for nursing education involves combating such misinformation by helping the potential participants understand the purpose of the seminar—what it is and what it is not—and outlining what will be expected of them. While it will not allay all anxiety, such preparation of nurses prior to entry into the seminar group seems to be useful in assisting them to understand what is expected of them and helping them use the experience more effectively. Generally, one session—either group or individual—seems sufficient. The same supportive preparation can be used in more advanced phases of the program to help the nurse therapist appreciate the importance of preparing patients for entry into group therapy.

The Didactic Seminar

The didactic seminar, which previously had been the first in the series, consists of 12 to 15 sessions of one and one-half to two hours a week. Content of the course encompasses the fundamentals of group psychotherapy. In general, sessions center around such topics as: the idea of group psychotherapy; group and therapist anxieties; individual identity and group situations; leadership and leadership styles; selection of patients; and administrative problems.

Previous educational objectives have been primarily cognitive in nature, revolving around acquisition and comprehension of knowledge. The current placement of this seminar permits more emphasis on the application and analysis of the content of the seminar. It further permits a bridge to be built between the cognitive and affective learning of the small group experience and the theoretical constructs deemed necessary for an individual to function as a group psychotherapist.

At one point, it was decided that the didactic seminar should be taught by discipline because of the disparity in both formal preparation and clinical experiences of the participants. Although the nurses participating in the first two phases of the seminary already have acquired specific knowledge in terms of terminology, classifications, and categories, they may be threatened by the use of the more universal abstractions, principles, and generalizations used by more sophisticated participants. Further, while the nurse may comprehend the material in terms of being able to translate and interpret, difficulties can arise in her understanding of implications and consequences. As she progresses through the program she does not seem to have any more significant difficulty than other trainees in terms of application, analysis, and synthesis of material. She may, however, have problems with evaluation—the ability to utilize material in making value judgements. Whatever her shortcomings, the nurse does bring to the seminar a rich array of clinical experiences not available to members of other disciplines. After evaluating the attempt to teach this phase of the program by discipline, both trainers and trainees decided that the differences in formal preparation and clinical experience among the trainees were complementary, thus adding to, rather than detracting from the seminar.

In keeping with findings reported by Lewin and his associates that certain methods of group discussion were superior to lecturing and individual instruction in changing ideas and affecting attitudes and experiences, the nurses evaluating methods of teaching used throughout the Center's program indicated the most effective learning experiences were those in which they had been active participants.[3] Role playing, group process exercises, or group discussions were considered most helpful. Films, followed by discussion, were seen as helpful; lectures were considered the least useful.

Supervised Experience as a Group Psychotherapist

Supervised training as a co-therapist must be preceded by completion of the first and second phases of the program. Whenever possible, the beginning nurse therapist is encouraged to observe the group (via a two-way mirror or closed-circuit television) for a period of four to six weeks and to attend supervisory sessions with those therapists currently in the group. Such observation permits the nurse therapist to learn about the structure, goals, and feelings of the group as well as allowing for some continuity of treatment. Supervision of all group therapists centers around patient-patient, patient-therapist, and therapist-therapist interactions. Countertransference problems of the therapist are examined and suggestions given with regard to these problems. As supervision progresses, the content matter of the group is de-emphasized and the use of group process in treatment is emphasized. Cognitive objectives emphasized include application, analysis, and synthesis.

Supervision is conducted on a weekly basis for a period of one year. After the first year, the therapist and supervisor are encouraged to meet regularly, the frequency of these meetings is determined according to the therapist's needs.

CLINICAL WORKSHOP. The demonstration group is led by an experienced group psychotherapist, and constitutes the final phase of the central program. Here the learning experiences include: (1) selection of a patient; (2) preparation of the patient for entrance into the group; and (3) beginning the development of the treatment contract. The seminar meets for two hours a week—one hour of observation followed by one hour of discussion. The participants observe the group from its first session through termination. If it becomes necessary for the patient to be seen individually in conjunction with group therapy, he will be followed by his nurse-trainee under the supervision of the group therapist. If the nurse has not had previous experience as an individual therapist, a rudimentary experience as an individual therapist is provided to build on at a later time.

While all of the stated objectives come into play during this seminar, synthesis and evaluation are stressed. This experience offers the nurse a forum to test her newly acquired skills in using materials more effectively and in making value judgments.

ELECTIVE CLINICAL WORKSHOPS. While elective clinical workshops are not included in the core preparation of a group psychotherapist, they are considered necessary in continuing his development and the sharpening of his skills. Generally, the workshops center around special application of psychotherapy—family therapy, crisis therapy, group therapy supervision, or more intensive development of specific techniques such as psychodrama. Sessions may be formal in that they are organized and scheduled by training staff, or they may arise spontaneously from the desire of therapists to learn from one another. As with most attempts at professional improvement, such seminars have full administrative approval.

CHARACTERISTICS OF NURSE TRAINEES

The trainees, particularly the nurse trainees, have characteristics similar to those that have been identified by Stien.[3] First, most of the nurses participating in the program are young, and while they do have experience in dealing with a variety of psychiatric patients, most of their work has been accomplished in the comparative security of an inpatient setting. Further, most of them lack experience with in-depth psychotherapeutic experience. At times, this lack has proved to be a handicap, often preventing them from seeing what was going on in the group. As a result of the lack of experience with individual patients, as well as a lack of experience in working with outpatients, some nurses became anxious when patients demonstrated possible psychotic or severe depressive symptoms. In general, such problems can be handled during the supervisory hour.

A second difficulty is getting the trainee to use the *group* in group psychotherapy. The therapist's tendency to deal with individual patients in the group instead of the group as a whole, may be due to inexperience, or it may be a manifestation of resistance to this method of treatment. Nurses, as well as other trainees, frequently believe group therapy is secondary to individual therapy. Regular supervision with an experienced group therapist seems to be the most effective method of overcoming this problem. The difficulty seems to be overcome more easily with trainees who have not had previous experience with individual therapy or who have been trained in an organization where group therapy is considered the treatment of choice rather than necessity.

A third difficulty encountered by a new nurse therapist is to allow herself to be drawn into the group when, in fact, the group could have functioned better without this intervention. The action-oriented nurse, finding herself in a position where she cannot *do*, may talk. Here again, regular supervision by a supervisor who observes the group routinely is useful.

CONCLUSION

Including the nurse in the interdisciplinary seminar is based on two premises: one, the nurse is a full member of the treatment team and therefore needs to be prepared to carry out treatment responsibilities; two, we recognize that definitions, principles, and techniques in group therapy are similar for all disciplines and are not unique to nursing. We believe that the uniqueness of the nurse in group therapy comes not from teaching her special techniques, and so on, but rather from the additional knowledge that nursing education and experience have made available to her.

As a member of the interdiciplinary training committee which recommends policy on who shall be trained, how they will be trained, and the limits of their utilization, the director of nursing education must be prepared to function as a liaison between nursing and the committee. She must also be prepared to function as a member of the interdisciplinary training team. In addition, she must offer additional preparation and support when necessary to nurses engaged in the program.

Although this paper has focused on the development of the nurse as a group psychotherapist, I have not meant to imply that that is the only expansion of her role. Other facets of the nurse's role at the Center include: individual, family, and couples therapy; home visits; crisis intervention; and consultation with community agencies. In short, as a full member of the treatment team, the nurse is prepared to carry the full range of responsibilities.

In an area such as the middle west, where there is a shortage of prepared nurse therapists, an organization must make a decision either to prepare nurses to engage in group psychotherapy or to exclude them. The administrative choice at the Western Missouri Mental Health Center has been to prepare them, and, the nurses at the Center rose to the challenge of accepting responsibility for learning.

Preparing nurses as group psychotherapists offers special problems because of the varying levels of educational preparation and clinical experience. A nurse with a master's degree may learn more quickly while a diploma school graduate may have to work the hardest in becoming a group psychotherapist. This may not always be the case, however. A willingness to invest in the preparation and extra support and to withstand the concern that all of the nurse trainees may not measure up to the trainees from other disciplines (and the ability to withstand the disappointment when they do not), are necessary ingredients for a successful program. We believe that developing and increasing the nurse's capacities is a worthwhile investment, not only to the nurse participants and to the agency, but to nursing as a profession.

REFERENCES

1. Mullan, H. and Rosenbaum M. Group Psychotherapy: Theory and Practice New York, The Free Press of Glencoe, 1962.
2. Lewin, K. Field Theory in Social Science. Cartwright, D., ed., New York, Harper & Row, Publishers, 1951.
3. Stien, A. The Training of the Group Psychotherapist. Rosenbaum, M., and Berger, M.M., eds., New York, Basic Books, Inc., 5th ed., 1963.

BIBLIOGRAPHY

A Committee of College and University Examiners. Bloom, B., ed. Taxonomy of Educational Objectives, London, Longmans, Green & Co. Ltd., 1st ed., 1956. Vol. 1.
Epps, R.L., Barnes, R., and McPartland, T.A. A Community Concern. Springfield, Ill., Charles C Thomas, Publisher, 1965.
Luft, J. Group Processes: An Introduction to Group Dynamics. Palo Alto, National Press Books, 9th ed., 1969.

DISCUSSION

Question:

We have had difficulty in instituting a process group because of the lack of adequately prepared trainers. How did you overcome this problem?

Mrs. Ramsburg:

The trainers for the group process seminar are members of our staff representing the disciplines of medicine, psychology, nursing and social work. I am one of the trainers. We were prepared for this specific role in a National Training Laboratory. We participate in the process seminars and the didactic sessions as well. The trainers alternate primary responsibility for a group of trainees in order to offer a variety of views. Other trainers are present and serve to clarify, validate, and offer other points of view.

Question:

As one of the interdisciplinary trainers, do you give the nurse trainees additional support? Do you meet with nurses "before and after" particular sessions?

Mrs. Ramsburg:

I meet with them before and I may meet with specific ones later, as the group progresses. Nurses often seek me out on their own, or if I hear or feel that one needs bolstering, I will approach her. It's my job to see that nurses are prepared and supported. Members of other disciplines meet with their people. This past year, any participant having particular difficulty in a group was able to work it out individually with the group trainer. I do not interfere with the group experience; however, I am available if the nurse needs support.

In our inpatient and outpatient services, group treatment is the major therapeutic mode carried out by the team of physicians, psychologists, social workers, and nurses. Some of the professional staff are prepared as group psychotherapists and some are not. In our rural area, there is a need for additional prepared therapists. Any registered nurse in the state interested and having potential, is eligible for selection to our group psychotherapy training program. My paper dealt with an interdisciplinary training program and describes those qualities unique to nursing which facilitate training and subsequent practice as a group psychotherapist in the *outpatient* service. We believe that our training program, which accepts nurses without degrees, has broad implications. There are many agencies that need help in initiating similar programs since there is an insufficient number of psychiatric nursing clinical specialists available.

We do not believe that all nurses or all psychiatrists or all psychologists or all

social workers can be group psychotherapists. We choose only those professionals we believe are interested and willing to assume responsibility for learning
and who demonstrated some potential in group treatment (not group therapy)
and those who demonstrate responsibility for planning patient care across service
area.

Question:

How do the other disciplines perceive the nurse group psychotherapist?

Mrs. Ramsburg:

For the past eight years we've had nurses running groups as co-therapists,
some as senior therapists. It is accepted that nurses function in this role. The
program and practice has evolved over a period of time. We made many
mistakes. One of the first seminars that I attended was totally disorganized and
in my opinion was a disaster. The evaluation confirmed that it was a disaster, but
the participants indicated they wanted to make it worth their time and effort.
The program I described evolved out of what people wanted. The nurses had a
choice whether or not to participate. They were willing to take the risk involved
in learning and in making mistakes. It was rough going and some of the nurses
pulled some real "boners." We went through a period of standing up and saying a
mistake was made and accepting responsibility. We had to stay out there and
prove we could do the job.

Question:

What is the rationale for separating the nurse supervisors from their nurse
supervisees in the interdisciplinary process seminars?

Mrs. Ramsburg:

In our present state system, nursing supervisors rate their supervisees
annually on an attitudinal scale which affects salary increments. We wanted to
avoid asking people to express themselves freely in a potentially problematic
situation. To insure fuller participation for all, we have supervisors rate
personnel but not their own supervisees.

Comment:

In the rural area in which I work, the problem is getting a group together.
We know that group therapy is a desirable approach. We cover many square
miles of territory and members of the group encounter problems of
transportation.

Comment:

We have a similar concrete problem in a small neighborhood where a mother can't get a babysitter or has no money for carfare. We do not have the resources to help her.

Comment:

In our community center we started prevention groups which are pretty primitive at this point. We'll select a core group and leave it open for clients to invite people they feel would be interest in participating with them.

Comment:

One of the things we did in a rural setting was to have a prevention group labeled "one-parent families." We offered baby-sitting services and transportation. As the group evolved, transportation became unnecessary because the mothers went by and picked each other up. The group really progressed because we offered a concurrent children's group, a pre-headstart program. It was one of the experiences I like to remember.

COMMUNITY INVOLVEMENT

Mental health problems can be a result of the individual and his interaction in his sociocultural environment. Despite the fact that causes of certain kinds of social pathology are well known, community mental health professionals are often unable to deal effectively with the sociopathological process. Moreover, health professionals know that the disadvantaged, especially, have not had access to nor have they been able to utilize mental health services. Conferees expressed an urgency to pursue and help clients seek and benefit from services and to identify and convert their needs into appropriate and effective demands for service. All too often the professionals' response results from community pressures, a fear of the explosive nature of the ghettos, and their own collective guilt. There is an increasing concern and action, however, on the part of mental health professionals who really care about reaching the lower socio-economic groups, particularly the population in the urban ghetto. What is needed is a climate which promotes learning about the community, its values and problems, which enourages nurses to participate in community action programs and which, most importantly, produces a system of health delivery that stands behind these commitments.

Nurses have worked in the community a long time, assuming among other roles that of patient advocate. The nurse's patient orientation, education, clinical experience, and general acceptance by the lower socioeconomic groups help to facilitate the nurse's contributions in community mental health more than those of other professionals. The nurse often works alone in sustaining the patient who is frequently caught in the power struggles in agencies, or between agencies and community groups, or both. Since mental health problems are so complex, nurses must join forces with other health disciplines and community groups in order to alter the system and bring about innovative changes.

Although traditional psychiatric nursing concepts, principles, and practice are necessary, we must be prepared to expand our roles, develop new theoretical frameworks, and acquire new skills in order to collaborate with the community and the client in more effective ways. The lessons to be learned are often painful and time consuming but must be learned if indeed we mean to engage the client in a productive relationship with his community.

One speaker emphatically cites that racism, as the number one mental health problem, greatly influences treatment. She hypothesizes that community mental health, as it exists in most places, is irrelevant and often destructive to black people. Basic to this hypothesis is the fact that decisions are often made for an about people without considering their needs or their life style. People are too easily labeled "sick" in view of their behavior, which, in reality, may be relevant to their style of life and the circumstances of the society they live in. Most people do not understand the nature and extent of racism that affects both blacks and whites. Learning about racism and oppression as mental health problems requires tremendous effort. As another speaker says, "People are able to liberate themselves of racist attitudes but it takes a lot of homework."

This chapter deals with the nurse's "homework." Changing the system means changing one's self and then trying to involve as many people as one can while still operating within the system. Conferees describe their collaboration and engagement with professionals, paraprofessionals, and clients in the systems in order to deal with feelings of apathy, isolation, deprivation, helplessness, and hopelessness. The authors describe the learning processes they went through as their nursing practice brought them face-to-face with the realities of a particular system such as the nursing system, the community mental health system, the client system, the local community or municipal, state, and federal government systems.

Community Mental Help In The City:
Are They Really "Patients?"

TONI M. FRANCIS, R.N., B.S., M.A.

INTRODUCTION

In November of 1968 I was assigned by the District of Columbia Public Health Department to a position as Mental Health Worker in a neighborhood health center in Washington. D.C. Prior to that time, I had worked as a clinical specialist in child psychiatric nursing at a community mental health center in the same area of the city, on a program for disturbed children and their families.

The population I served, and continue to serve, is predominantly poor and black. The great majority of them must depend on the U.S. Congress, through federal and city agencies, for their income, food supply, housing, health care, education, employment, and protection. In all areas the resources available to them are woefully inadequate.* Those who attempt to fulfill their needs outside

*According to a U.S. Government Printing Office pamphlet, *We the Black People of the United States*, (U.S. G.P.O., 19690-338-305), the Negro median income is 59 percent of the white. Black people are twice as likely as white to be out of work and one in three black workers is unemployed or seriously underemployed. Of the black population, 14 percent are on welfare, as compared with 3 percent for whites. The most recent surveys published by the U.S. Census Bureau, reported that, in 1967, the average life expectancy for black people was 64.6 years; 71.3 for whites (U.S., H.E.W., National Center for Health Statistics, *Vital Statistics of the U.S.*, 1967, Vol. II, Life Tables). The infant mortality rate was 35.9 percent for black babies; 19.7 percent for white babies (U.S., H.E.W., National Center for Health Statistics, *The Monthly Vital Statistics Report*, 1967, Vol. XVII, No.

the governmental system are met with the well-publicized problems of slum landlords, high food prices for substandard produce, rising costs of private medical care and schooling, scarcity of jobs that guarantee a living wage, and an alarming increase in crime of which they are most often the victims.

I soon realized that I had a lot to learn in my new position as Mental Health Worker. In the following pages I will attempt to articulate what I have learned and how it has shaped my professional role.

MENTAL HEALTH—WHAT IT IS NOT

Although psychiatrists in this country probably would deny it, their classification of psychopathology is based in the main on cultural norms. It is good to have a steady job; it is bad to conceive out of wedlock; it is good to obey the law; it is bad to be suspicious. In each case, one could substitute "healthy" for "good," and "unhealthy" for "bad." Psychoanalytic theory and therapy, on which psychiatry is based, were modeled on a white, middle- and upper-middle-class Victorian society. Psychiatry defined behavior in terms of the moral values which predominated then, as they do now, in our society. In short, psychiatry attempted to base its definitions of emotional health and illness on a standard deviation which found conformists healthy and everyone else "sick."

Granted, there are some diagnostic entities—described, labeled, and treated by psychiatrists—that apparently exist cross-culturally such as unconscious depression, the schizophrenias, and others. It is not within the scope of this paper to attempt an exhaustive appraisal of the entire nosology of psychiatric disorders. However, there are several areas where I find the established classification useless when it is applied to black people. Emotional illness must be redefined in terms of an individual's life experiences, needs, value systems, and culture.

Unfortunately, most analyses—and the list of studies is lengthy—attempt to fit black people into pre-existing conceptual frameworks that are inapplicable. It is like trying to push a square peg through a round hole but it is not child's play.

---

12). Statistics on housing, on education as it relates to income, and on crime and its victims show similar differences between races. The National Urban League, which issued comparable figures in, *Cold Facts*, compiled for the year, 1968, noted: more than 40% of the 22 million Black Americans are poor; i.e., earn less that $4,000 per year per family; that the reading level among Black students is three years below that of average White students; that three out of ten Black families live in substandard housing, as compared to one in ten White families; and that of every 100 infant deaths, 75% are Black (Published in *Muhammed Speaks*, July 18, 1969, official paper of the Muslims). With respect to employment among Black men in Washington, D.C. . . . Liebow states, ". . . a man who is able and willing to work cannot earn enough to support himself, his wife, and one or more children. . .". (Liebow, E., *Tally's Corner*, Boston, Little Brown and Company, 1967, pp. 50-51).

All the ill-conceived efforts to explain away the "problem" of the black man in this country have only succeeded in reinforcing the conviction among both blacks and whites that there is something innately wrong with black people; in other words, that they are an inferior race, that their problems are due to low intelligence, laziness, hypersexuality, an antisocial—even violent—character, and overaggressiveness. Sound familiar? It should. It is the common stereotype applied to black people in this nation.

The destruction extends beyond reinforcement of racist attitudes. In the name of mental health and humanitarianism, white "missionaries" have removed scores of black children from their "unfit" parents. Frequently, the white "missionary" has never seen the family at home and has not even attempted to weigh the positive aspects in the family's life against the certain damage of separation.*

Sometimes the destruction is more subtle, but nevertheless effective. Thousands of young black boys are labeled antisocial, aggressive, acting-out, impulsive, or sociopathic when they express their outrage at the violence being done to them and to their families each day. These children then are subjected to psychiatric "treatment" aimed at coercing them to "adjust" to a society which says that white is good and black is bad. Grier and Cobbs, both Black psychiatrists, describe the "Black Norm" as follows;

> For his (the Black man's) own survival . . . he must develop a cultural paranoia *in which every white man is a potential enemy unless proved otherwise* . . . .
> *He develops a sadness and intimacy with misery which has become a characteristic of Black Americans. It is a* cultural depression *and a* cultural masochism.
> . . . .
> *He can never quite respect laws which have no respect for him, and laws designed to protect white men are viewed as white men's laws . . . The result may be described as a* cultural anti-socialism, *but it is simply an accurate reading of one's environment.*[2]

Add to these the brilliant observation of Black psychoanalyst, Frantz Fanon:

> *A close study (of the psychology of the black man) should be divided into two parts:*
> 1. *a psychoanalytic interpretation of the life experience of the black man;*
> 2. *a psychoanalytic interpretation of the Negro myth.*[3]

It must be clear by now that much of psychiatric theory is irrelevant in defining the psychological situation of black people in this country. This is true,

*Malcolm X's description of his own family's disintegration is a case in point. Haley, A. (ed.). *The Autobiography of Malcolm X.* New York, Grove Press, Inc., 1965, pp. 17-19.

of course, in any country where black people are oppressed, and, having discovered this, I had to search for a new conceptual framework and redefine my goals. Grier and Cobbs offered some direction:

> Clinicians who are interested in the psychological functioning of black people must get acquainted with this body of character traits which we call the Black Norm. It is a normal complement of psychologoical devices, and to find the amount of sickness a black man has, one must first total all that appears to represent illness and then subtract the Black Norm. What remains is illness and a proper subject for therapeutic endeavor. To regard the Black Norm as pathological and attempt to remove such traits by treatment would be akin to analyzing away a hunter's cunning or a banker's prudence. . . .
> . . . Too much of psychotherapy involves striving only for a change in the inner world and a consequent adaptation to the world outside. Black people cannot abide this and thoughtful therapists know it. A black man's soul can live only if it is oriented toward a change of the social order. A good therapist helps a man change his inner life so that he can more effectively change his outer world.[4]

Let us look now at the inner life and the outer world of the black man in this country.

OPPRESSION AND RACISM

This nation of ours values things over people. I consider that a truism, though many would dispute me. I will not attempt to justify the statement here, except to point out that the U.S. expends the majority of its wealth on things, especially weapons. This, presumably, makes it the most powerful nation on earth. But the wealth and power are concentrated in the hands of a few, while millions are denied even the bare essentials of life.

There was a time when this country numbered black people among its "things," and justified such economic oppression by defining black people as less than human. Even the U.S. Constitution defines a slave as three-fifths of a human being.[5] Slavery has been abolished—on paper—but the definition of black people as subhuman; as "nigger savages," to use Fanon's phrase, has continued to the present.[6] What began as a rationalization for economic exploitation has endured in the form of racial prejudice.

Racism, for the purpose of this paper, is the operational hatred of black people.* The word "operational" is important here for two reasons. First, while racism may exist only on the unconscious level, it is reflected nevertheless in behavior that conforms to racist attitudes and beliefs. Second, there is no such thing as black racism because racism presupposes the power to exploit others

---

* This definition was contributed by Dr. W. Augustus L. Reid, Psychiatrist, Children's Program, Area C Community Mental Health Center, Washington, D.C.

and black people have no power in this country. Their tendency to sterotype and to hate "Whitey" in a collective fashion is a normal reaction to the dehumanizing oppression to which white society has subjected them.

Let me make myself very clear. When I speak of white people, I am not necessarily referring to white skin and Caucasian features. I am speaking of people who have incorporated the attitudes of racism into their functioning personalities and who, therefore, support institutionalized racism. Whether or not they are capable of personal racist acts is another question. To quote Fanon again:

> The Negro problem does not resolve itself into the problem of Negroes living among white men but rather of Negroes exploited, enslaved, despised by a colonialist, capitalist society that is only accidentally white.[7]

Many people of color have incorporated racist attitudes also and the enabling psychological defense mechanism of identification with the oppressor (a survival technique) has been well documented and described.[8] It is also true that people with white skin are capable of ridding themselves of most, if not all, racist attitudes, but the process is a slow and painful one and they risk alienation and ostracism from society at large.

How then does racism operate? Essentially, it works in two ways. The first is through systematic indoctrination of all people in this country to believe that white is superior and black is inferior. The black child hears his parents—who were themselves thoroughly indoctrinated—depreciate "niggers" and talk about how smart the white man is. On television, in comic books, through white dolls and bad cowboys with black hats, through white angels and black devils, white lies and black magic, a white Santa Claus, and a white God, black children learn that black is bad. This bad feeling about themselves is reinforced at home, in school, on the streets, in church, by all the communications media and every institution.

Recall for a moment a basic tenet of psychiatric theory: at the root of all functional mental disorders lies a negative self-image. Yet every black person in this country is taught to hate himself—from the cradle on. Hence, racism intrudes itself into his developing personality and, in most instances, results in the psychological destruction of his ego by age four.[9]

I have already alluded to the second way in which racism operates and that is through the external force of oppression. Poussaint says, "The feeling that one can have "control" over social forces is crucial to one's feelings of ego strength and self-esteem,"[10],*

---

*Incidentally, oppression or exploitation is not limited to Black people in this country. According to Dr. Thomas Levin of The Einstein Medical College in New York. "There are five underclasses in this country; non-whites, the poor, the young, the old, and women." (Talk presented to the staff, Area C Community Mental Health Center, Washington, D.C., 1969).

In fact, racism is institutionalized in this country. A capitalistic society must exploit large numbers of people in order to amass its great wealth. This exploitation is made possible initially through violence and terrorism, such as that inflicted on the black slaves our forefathers brought from Africa. The threat of violence still hangs in the air and we have seen it erupt when the established order was threatened. Recent examples are the "police riot" in Chicago during the Democratic national convention of 1968 and the assaults on members of the Black Panther Party in that city and in Los Angeles.[11] But more covert forms of subjugation are also at work.

> In Capitalist societies the educational system, whether lay or clerical, the structure of moral reflexes handed down from father to son, the exemplary honesty of workers who are given a medal after fifty years of good and loyal service and the affection which springs from harmonious relations and good behavior—all these aesthetic expressions of respect for the established order serve to create around the exploited person an atmosphere of submission and inhibition which lightens the task of policing considerably.[12,13]

But the problem of racism is more pervasive even than this. Witness the treatment of Bobby Seale, a defendant in the infamous "Chicago Eight Trial." He was denied legal counsel of his choice. Serious questions have arisen about the impartiality of the judge and many technical issues remain unresolved. The spectacle of such injustice perpetrated in the name of justice makes a mockery of this country's constitutional guarantee of equal protection under the law.

I have already cited statistics which reflect the failure of this country to provide for the health, education, and social welfare of black people, especially in comparison with the white population.

According to Grier and Cobbs, in this "Christian" land, even the Churches support the racist system and have helped to maintain the submissive position of black people.

> Religion plays a role in the cancer of black self-depreciation and the exaltation of whites. . . . Religion teaches that one should in general be kind, be fair, be modest, restrain impulses, and love everyone.
> It is designed to evoke guilt. . . .
> An initial assumption of guilt, if taken seriously, may or may not cripple white Americans, but it is lethal to black men. . . .
> The result is the pious, white, freshly laundered Negro, sans dirt, sans sins, and sans soul.[14]

Finally, the mass media, by selective and biased reporting have failed to keep the people of the U.S. informed. Newspapers, radio, and television extol the virtues of capitalism to a largely uncritical audience. They have consistently presented black leaders, who have championed the rights of their people, as violent, subversive men. The notable exception is Dr. Martin Luther King, who was widely tolerated because he preached nonviolence. Make no mistake; I neither like nor advocate violence. But there is a gross contradiction in this nation; on the one hand, it condemns black leaders for their alleged violence; on the other hand, this country was conceived in violence, maintains its power through violence, and has built into its every institution violence against a large segment of its own citizenry. I refer to the more than 22 million black Americans. The sad truth is that most people understand neither the nature nor the extent of racism in this country.

> What we are discovering in short is that the United States . . . is a racist society in a sense and to a degree that we have refused so far to admit, much less face . . . The tragedy of race relations in the United States is that there is no American Dilemma. White Americans are not torn and tortured by the conflict between their devotion to the American Creed and their actual behavior. They are upset by the current state of race relations, to be sure. But what troubles them is not that justice is being denied but that their peace is being shattered and their business interrupted.[15]

In summary, black people in this country are psychologically and physically assaulted on all sides. These external pressures, superimposed on an already negative self-image, create among black Americans a population "at high risk" in terms of community mental health.

THE OTHER SIDE OF THE COIN

Unfortunately, what I have presented thus far is only one side of the coin. On the other side are the psychologically damaging effects of racism among white people. The process through which racist attitudes are inculcated in black people, parallels the process in white people. Originally, the characterization of the black man as sub-human was, of course, an attempt on the part of our slave-owning ancestors to justify their economic oppression of slaves. Cleaver describes it graphically in *Soul on Ice:*

> The Omnipotent Administrator (White man) conceded to the Supermasculine Menial (Black man) all of the attributes of masculinity associated with the Body: strength, brute power, muscle, even the beauty of the brute body. Except one—sex.[16]

He goes on to say that the white man thereby attempted to deny the black man access to the white woman. But it is impossible to separate sex from the body. The stereotype took firm hold and the black myth to this day includes the belief that black men excel in sexual performance.

To put it another way, the white man denied and repressed his own sexual and aggressive drives—unacceptable according to the Puritan ethic—and projected them onto the black man who became sterotyped as "Evil personified." Thus the white man attempted to rationalize his oppression of the black man by defining him as savage. Obviously, this psychological exercise backfired on the white man who was left with deep-seated conflicts about his sexual and aggressive drives; with an irrational fear of the black race as violent; with hatred of the black man as his sexual superior; and with unresolved guilt feelings stemming from his unconscious drives and his cruel treatment of black people. Moreover, the white man deprived himself of knowledge and experience of another culture and of satisfying relationships with black people. He has emerged alienated from his own body and emotions; separated by a wall of prejudice from his black brother. Something is drastically wrong when a man who would not think of kicking his cat, would not hesitate to lynch a "nigger." Most white people do not realize the extent to which they are manipulated by a powerful, elite clique because they have swallowed the lie that they are superior beings. Hence, they are duped and unaware of their own oppression.

Needless to say, racism exacts a terrible price among both black and white in the U. S. The problem of racism from the point of view of mental health is staggering, and its effects, monstrous. How, where, and with whom does one attempt to intervene when the task seems so overwhelming? Perhaps a partial answer may be suggested as I describe the rationale that guides me in my practice.

ARE THEY REALLY "PATIENTS?"

One of the basic principles that guides my practice is this statement by Fanon: "A normal Negro child, having grown up within a normal family, will become abnormal on the slightest contact with the white world."[17] As I have pointed out, that abnormality will consist in the fact of his blackness with all that it connotes in this white society. He will immediately, ". . . be confronted by the dilemma, *turn white or disappear*."[18] But, Fanon continues:

> *He should be able to take cognizance of a possibility of existence. In still other words, if society makes difficulties for him because of his color, if in his dreams I establish the expression of an unconscious desire to change color, my objective will not be that of dissuading him from it by advising him to 'keep his place;' on the contrary, my objective, once his motivations have been brought into consciousness, will be to put him in a position to* choose *action (or passivity) with respect to the real source of the conflict—that is, toward the social structures.*[19]

In line with this, one of my primary responsibilities is to sort out for myself, and my client, how much his difficulties are caused by this oppressive society and how much he contributes by his own intrapsychic pathology. The latter will undoubtedly also reflect this racist society as it has been incorporated into his personality. Hence, I have a continuing responsiblity to educate myself and my clients about the pathogenic environment in which we live.*

To illustrate what this means in practical terms, I will present clinical material from one of my case records.

Mr. and Mrs. X live in a public housing apartment in a poor, Black neighborhood. I saw them jointly for several months in weekly marital counseling sessions. Mrs. X related during an interview that she had been quite upset over an incident the previous week. She and her teenage daughter had been terrified by a White man peering in their window at night. She had called the local police, who apprehended the man and brought him to her home for positive identification. The two White policemen asked her what to charge him with and then intimated that she was having an affair with the man. When she was summoned to a preliminary hearing, she had to wait several hours before the policemen arrived, whereupon she was informed that she would be notified when to appear in court. That was several months ago. Mrs. X still has not been called to appear in court, and in spite of several inquiries, has been unable to obtain any information about the case.

When Mrs. X first related this incident to me, I responded that a Black man peering in someone's window at night in a White suburban community would have been charged immediately and, in all probability, would have been clapped behind bars under prohibitive bail. The insulting intimation that the woman had been having an illicit affair with the stranger would not have been made or, if it had, the police officer would also have been charged. My point in making these remarks was to illustrate for Mrs. X in a very personal way, how this society discriminates against Black people, not only in individual Black-White encounters, but also through its official institutions, in this instance the Judicial system. I suggested to Mrs. X that she seek legal assistance. This particular couple has had continuing difficulty with mutual distrust. The incident cited above, unfortunately, increased Mr. X's suspicions. I will have more to say about that later.

The situation of Mr. and Mrs. X also illustrates the interaction of intrapsychic pathology and societal pathology. For example, Mr. X is given to explosive outbursts of anger, especially when he has been drinking. In fact, this was his wife's chief complaint when she first sought mental health services. A look at her husband's past history reveals that he was incarcerated for "aggressive," "antisocial" behavior between the ages of 16 and 22. Upon his release, he encountered repeated difficulties with the police who apprehended him several times on vague charges. In one instance the judge who presided at his hearing found the charges so absurd that he laughed openly in court.

*Actually, the ability to distinguish sick person from sick society presupposes a thorough understanding of both individual psychopathology and of the pathogenic society.

Nevertheless, he sentenced Mr. X to 30 days in jail, knowing that the latter had a wife and five children. Needless to say, Mr. X was thereby denied the ability to provide for and protect his family, which is the essence of masculinity in our society.

As a child, Mr. X had been told repeatedly by his Mother and other significant adults that he was "bad" and "evil." His subsequent treatment by legal and judicial agents reinforced his already damaged self-concept. Such incidents as his 30-day confinement have left him in severe psychological conflict.

Had he the opportunity to direct his anger outward at its source, the society which oppresses him, he could thereby discharge that anger in a psychologically healthy manner. This would be normal, adaptive behavior. But as a Black man in a White society, which has labeled him dangerous and violent, unable to afford the services of an interested and concerned lawyer, Mr. X is impotent. If he had known that free legal services are available through the Neighborhood Legal Services Program which is funded by the Office of Economic Opportunity, he *might* have been able to fight these convictions. Like most poor, Black people, however, he is ill-informed about such resources.

Hence, Mr. X directs his anger inward upon himself, and this attempt to cope with it is facilitated by his poor self-image. As a result, he turns to drinking to escape his depressing situation and as an opportunity for cathartic outbursts of rage which give him an artificial feeling of power. This maladaptive behavior creates serious problems in his family relationships.

Damaged self-concept among Black males is a psychological problem that I have encountered repeatedly in my work. It can be traced to slavery days when Black women disciplined their male children harshly because they knew that any Black man who opposed the White master was "committing suicide." The situation today is essentially the same. The Black woman is torn by conflict between wanting her man to survive and wanting him to stand up like a man. Most often the conflict is unconscious so that she is unaware of her ambivalence and does not understand the Black man's objections to her behavior.

This problem is compounded by the self-hatred which I alluded to before. Black people in our society learn to hate themselves and they often project that unconscious hatred onto other people of color. Many identify with the oppressor—the White man—in a desperate and futile attempt to escape their Blackness. The direct result is mistrust among them and this gives rise to enormous difficulties in Black male-female relationships.

It was my responsibility to explain to Mr. and Mrs. X the interplay between intrapsychic and societal forces which I have just described and to relate this to the problems they experience in family life. There are many other aspects to this case which contribute to the disharmony in their lives—overcrowding and lack of privacy, physical health problems, meager income, a terribly inadequate school system, a neighborhood terrorized by frequent and serious crimes, and so on.

It should be clear by now that traditional psychiatric theory and techniques cannot be applied to Black people. A psychiatric professional who attempts to work from the traditional model with Black people is not only irrelevant, but often destructive. If I were leading from that position, I would no doubt find a great deal of intrapsychic pathology among my clients. I would tend to see their normal adaptive reactions to racism and oppression as symptoms of psychiatric illness, and I would then launch into a "treatment program" which is doomed to failure at the outset. But what is worse, I would be labeling healthy people sick, stigmatizing and perhaps even hospitalizing them, when the illness lies not in them, but in society.

Fortunately, I was able to perceive the irrelevance of traditional psychiatry in the context of mental health among Black people and to define the behavior and experiences of Black people in terms of the racist society in which we live.

The rest, as they say, is history. The other important principles that guide my practice are already familiar and have been discussed extensively elsewhere on both the theoretical and clinical levels. From nursing education I achieved awareness of the whole man, with all his needs, fears, and desires: from psychiatry I learned the significance of a trusting relationship as the primary vehicle through which constructive change occurs; from child psychiatry I took on the firm convictions that parent-child relationships are pivotal and that prevention is the hope of the future; and from community mental health I became aware of the dynamic interdependence between the individual and his community. But the learning that has been most relevant to my practice is not found in any established curriculum, and that is my growing understanding of racism and oppression as mental health problems in this country and particularly in relation to my clientele.

But I wonder—are they really "patients?"

GENERAL REFERENCES

1. Malcolm X. The Autobiography of Malcolm X. With the Assistance of Haley, A. New York, Grove Press, Inc., 1965, pp. 17-19.
2. Grier, W. H. and Cobbs, P. M. Black Rage. New York, Basic Books, Inc. 1968. p. 149.
3. Fanon, F. Black Skin, White Masks. New York, Grove Press, Inc., 1967, p. 151.
4. Grier and Cobbs, op. cit., pp. 150-151.
5. Constitution of the United States, Article I, Section 2, para. 3.
6. Fanon, op. cit., p. 199.
7. Ibid., p. 202.
8. Grier and Cobbs, op. cit., p. 166-167.
9. Arieti, S. ed. The American Handbook of Psychiatry, New York, Basic Books, Inc. 1966. Vol. III, p. 639

10. Poussaint, A. F. The Negro American: His Self-Image and Integration, *In* Barbour, F. B., ed., The Black Power Revolt. Porter Sargent, 1968, p. 98.
11. Levin, T. Talk presented to staff, Area C Community Mental Health Center, Washington, D.C., 1969.
12. Walker, D. Rights in Conflict: Convention Week in Chicago, August 25-29, 1968. New York, E. P. Dutton & Co., Inc., 1969.
13. Fanon, F. The Wretched of the Earth. New York, Grove Press, Inc., 1968, p. 38.
14. See Kozol, J. Death at an Early Age. Boston, Houghton Mifflin Company, 1967, for a description of racism as it operates in public schools.
15. Grier and Cobbs, op. cit., pp. 65-66.
16. Silberman, C. E. Crisis in Black and White. New York, Vintage Books, 1964, pp. 9-10.
17. Cleaver, E. Soul on Ice. New York, McGraw-Hill Book Company, 1968, p. 162.
18. Fanon, op. cit., p. 143.
19. Ibid., p. 100.
20. Ibid.

DISCUSSION

Question:

Acceptance by the black people in your community is the prerequisite for sound nursing practice. What steps are required in the development of acceptance? Would you describe what you did, what you thought, what you felt, and what relationship was developed with the larger, white system?

Miss Francis:

My graduate education and clinical experiences were primarily in a poor black area in New York City. I became very interested in problems of poverty in the inner city and, following graduation, thinking that I knew something about it, I took a position in a community mental health center in Washington, D.C.

I soon realized that I really didn't understand what clients were saying. I really didn't identify with them. I couldn't empathize with their position—I didn't understand what their living situation was like and so on. Not knowing how to handle my reactions or the situation, I stayed pretty much behind those protective walls of the center and let the clients come to me.

When I was assigned as a mental health worker in a neighborhood clinic, I viewed this as an opportunity to get closer to the clients, to find out more about their life style, and to explore my feelings. I realized I was not meeting their needs and therefore my practice was not relevant. I was operating pretty much under the traditional psychiatric model. As I moved into the role of mental health worker, I found myself alone and unprotected. I realized that I had a tremendous amount to learn and I started reading—*Soul On Ice, Autobiography of Malcolm X, Manchild in the Promised Land, Wretched of the Earth*—the books that acquaint you with the black experience in a white society. I began to talk a great deal with my black colleagues and my black clients in order to identify feelings. I started attending community meetings, trying to identify problems they were trying to cope with. As a result, I met many members of the community, became involved in their work, and I learned a great deal about the issues important to them.

As clients came to know me, they began to call me and I would get reports from neighbors about a family which was of concern to them. I would be contacted by school personnel, a settlement house, by a raft of agencies in the neighborhood, the welfare department, the police, the courts, and my fellow staff members at the clinic—the calls came from all over.

When I receive a report about a family, I request that the family be alerted to the fact that I am at the clinic and to please call me if they wish to talk with me. I believe it is important that they indicate an interest in receiving help. Usually they call, saying, "I have a problem." Later, we sit down in my office or in their home, and talk about their problems—what are their most immediate needs and how can we begin to meet those needs. For example, a mother will come in with a child. The problem is the child, as she sees it. The child may be a truant from school or is getting into fights on the street, or the child is a bed-wetter. We talk about how the child expresses the problem; how and when did it start; how the child describes or explains the behavior. Usually, if I can, I will see the child at home with the parent. Invariably, the problem is in getting to know how the family operates. Generally, the problem is between the parents. I get involved with the parental relationship as well as child-rearing issues. I become available to them—a person they can call on when needs arise.

It is mainly through close, personal relationships with colleagues and clients that one develops awareness of what is going on in society and how black people are affected. I redefined my role because the old psychiatric traditional model simply didn't fit. Two major responsibilities in mental health work are identifying human needs and assisting people in meeting them, and trying to share with people about the circumstances they find themselves in—why they feel the way they do, and so on.

How the client uses this information is really up to him. Some of them join social organizations in an attempt to change their mode of living and that of their black brothers and sisters; some move out of the depressive cycle because they can see themselves as not at fault, not the cause of all these difficulties, and direct their anger appropriately toward the source.

I have learned a great deal from some professionals who work with me on a part-time basis in the neighborhood. I found that they can move in and work very effectively because they have lived the experience of the clients. They did not have to go through this reorientation process. I find it extremely difficult however, to criticize a black person on my team who is in error as it is difficult for me to be called a racist by a black person. You know, it's very subtle the way racism operates in us, black and white. I notice, for example, that I am more challenging with white people than I am with black people. It's going to take more work and readjustment of my thinking and feelings and attitudes before I can deal similarly with black and white. Perhaps I'll never reach that point, but this is the way racism operates.

We have been self-protective, following the physician rather than really looking at what is needed. What *is* mental health, and how can nursing make a contribution? We have supported the status quo rather than operate aggressively in changing the system.

I started to work in a community; you find out more about the system and become part of the system. It is essential to become a part of the community; it is the only effective way to work. The fact that this, in turn, alienates me from the larger system—the employing system, the larger white societal system—is really out of my hands.

Comment:

It's a two-way street! I believe there is a need to work through the larger system as well as the community. Your attitude concerns me! What does one do to cause growth in the larger systems? You can influence the system. You win a few and you lose a few through the process of aggression. For example, in the field service I work in, the issue of diagnosis became a problem. We're the only group related to the mental health center that writes at the bottom of the diagnostic category "no diagnosis," because we don't diagnose anybody. We had to fight for that. Another example: the majority of our second-year residents were white and the field workers were black. We meet with the residents each week as the doctors take care of the medical problems; in other words, they write the prescriptions and see the patients for psychiatric re-evaluation and medication. We work as a team and if there's an emergency in the home, the resident goes out with the field worker. We had to exert tremendous pressure to get the residents out of the center. There is a great deal of reticence, so one goes through a process of working with them on their level saying, "You have something to gain in this experience as well as supporting the field worker in the delivery of care."

Miss Francis:

As I mentioned, there are nine people who work with me on a part-time basis. We call them neighborhood mental health workers as opposed to the people who remain in the confines of the community mental health center. In another section of the city, there is a similar group; totally, there are several dozen of us who work in the neighborhood. We feel that we are the people who have the expertise, who understand what is needed in terms of mental health in the black community. We have offered to meet with the people of the center who are interested in finding out more about the black community and about working as mental health workers in the black community. They are free to come to our meetings to discuss what they would be interested in doing on a team to provide relevant mental health services. A number do come to the meetings, discuss with us what they would like to do, and in which area of the city they would like to work. We encourage them if we feel they can offer relevant service, and then they are absorbed into one of the teams working in the neighborhood. If we feel they are in need of additional learning, and changing attitudes, we refer them back to what we call, "the caucuses."

There are two groups, one black and one white; we participate in both. Individuals get together with members of their own races to examine their attitudes in regard to racial problems. This has been going on for several months. Obviously, there are many people on the staff of the community mental health center who do not respond to either of these attempts to share what we have learned, to work on attitudes, to prepare people to work more effectively. A number of people at the community mental health center have resigned. A number of them are still fighting us because they see us as a power group, trying to usurp their authority, which, of course, is unfortunate. It is a continuing process and we are working on it.

The reason we take a fairly aggressive position is that we have seen too many cases where a family or a person was destroyed in the psychological sense and, to some extent in the physical sense, in the name of mental health. So we have something to protect. For example, separating children from their families or hospitalizing people unnecessarily. If a center cannot come to grips with the racial issue in its own community, then it is unqualified to move as a united body into the black community, or Puerto Rican community, or any other minority group living in the same geographical area. We must make personnel understand that it is devastating to bring a mother into the hospital, give her 400 milligrams of thorazine a day, and say, "When you don't hear voices any longer you go home, rest and don't worry about feeding your babies or how you are going to pay your rent."

Comment:

Coming from the deep south, my orientation has been the psychiatric nurse treats the psychiatric patient in a one-to-one relationship or in groups of various sorts. However, many problems don't fit the traditional framework. In many cases, there just isn't anybody to do what needs to be done and so I have asked myself, "Can we stop?" Do we limit our concern, activities, and our interests? I believe we must go out and do more and get into other areas. I try this and I try that, and I get so frustrated! Then I say, "I'll go out and fight." So far, it's been muddling along, without much direction, not much support, but I feel definitely supported from this group of mental health nurses.

Comment:

You know, I really question whether it's a problem of trying to decide where we end. I think the problem is to decide where we begin. Traditional psychiatry has become engaged in a process of exclusion. Problems are taken out of the community to be put into the hospital; or to identify "patients;" or to come to the community mental health center, or whatever.

The reverse of that is to be inclusive. The problems have to be included in the community they exist in; this means becoming involved where the problem exists. You become engaged in a process with the patient in his social system, identify what the problems are and resolve them together. Mental health workers do not have the answers and we cannot tell the school system what they're doing wrong or tell the family what they're doing wrong. The questions we face are: do we alientate ourselves from our system; do we alienate the patient from his system? I think that is one of the greatest challenges.

There is always the danger of alienation. The dilemma is how to carry out the transactions between the agency and the community or the agency and other agencies without provoking alienation. This is very important—it is a negotiation process!

It has been said that nurses are in a better position than any other discipline to bridge the gap. To say that any one professional bridges the gap is a myth. What bridges the gap is the negotiation process.

Comment:

As a nurse, I am not as threatening as our social worker or our psychologist to the county commissioner whom we depend on for money. Does less threatening mean less power? It does mean less power, and you don't change the system overnight but over a five-year period I've seen changes take place as a result of what nurses can do, not because of the power that they have.

Question:

In our particular society most of us internalize prejudice against the black and white. Is there a danger in identifying too much with the subculture so that we lose objectivity?

Miss Francis:

There has been a study done that found that those mental health people who identified most closely with the clients were the most effective in bringing about constructive change in the clients. When we talk about objectivity and not getting involved, this is a "distance maneuver" for safety, which actually keeps us from being useful to clients. When we focus on "*I'm* the therapist" and "*he's* the patient," it's a mistake.

I feel a great sense of urgency and a sense of fear. We'll sit around and talk about issues and we'll all go home to our own centers, to the same setting, and do the same thing.

I can envision what is happening between white and black, between the young and the establishment. I see a fairly immediate violent confrontation, unless we get involved and are able to do something about it. After all, we're supposed to understand how people feel, how they interact, how they operate, something about psychological dynamics and sociological problems which we don't understand in ourselves in terms of our attitudes. Yet we're trying to change the attitudes of other people who have a tremendous amount of influence on a great numbers of lives. How can we possibly beat that clock, change the system in time to avoid violent destructive confrontation?

The Role of the Nurse in Consultation and Education to Community Caretakers

JUDITH ANNE MARTOIS, R.N., M.S.

Federal legislation, designed to combat mental illness and mental retardation, and initiated in 1963, brought about a new approach involving the nationwide development of a broad array of preventive, diagnostic, outpatient and inpatient treatment facilities, and rehabilitative, educative and consultative services in the community. A distinctive feature of the new approach is that the programs are local, community-centered, and immediately available.[1] California's plan for developing community-centered, programs to deal with a growing mental health problem was approved by the state legislature in 1957, namely, by the Short-Doyle Act for Community Mental Health Services.[2]

The Los Angeles County Department of Mental Health was formed in 1960 under the Short-Doyle Act. In the first year, the Department had a total staff allocation of six positions, a budget of one million dollars, and a beginning preventive program of professional mental health consultation to community agencies. By July 1, 1968, the Department had grown to 308.5 allocated positions, a 19.9 million dollar budget, nine Regional Service Offices, a Day Treatment Center and jointly operated programs with the County Departments of Health, Hospitals, and Probation. Because California's 1967 Lanterman-Petris-Short Legislation placed more new responsibilities on participating California counties and cities, including the establishment of psychiatric emergency teams as well as the screening process for all voluntary and involuntary requests for admission to state hospitals, the Department was given authorization to expand to 552.5 allocated positions, and a gross budget for local programs of approximately 30.6 million dollars for the 1969-1970 fiscal year. All of this is in addition to 22 million dollars authorized to maintain state hospital inpatient care for Los Angeles County through a contract between the county and state.[3] Los Angeles County has the largest population of all California counties, and expends approximately $1.75 per capita on its mental health program.[4] The 30 million dollars allocated for local services may be contrasted to the more than 100 million dollars allocated for local services in New York City.[5]

The setting for this paper in the San Gabriel Valley Mental Health Service, one of nine regional services of the Los Angeles County Department of Mental Health. Much has been written about the role of the nurse in the community mental health center, and publications have concentrated on the functions of the nurse with regard to direct service to patient, for example, the nurse as a psychotherapist, the supportive role of the nurse, and the individual versus community orientation of nurses.[6-8] There is an acute need for assessing at what level nurses are prepared to function effectively and accept treatment responsibilities on a peer level with other mental health personnel. Another vital function of nursing in community mental health (and the one with which this paper is concerned), is that of mental health consultation and education—clearly the preventive aspects of community mental health.

CATCHMENT AREA

The San Gabriel Valley catchment area is the most populous service area in Los Angeles County with 1,500,000 residents; it contains populations of the highly affluent as well as ghetto dwellers. The area also has five health districts, 26 cities of diverse characteristics, 33 school districts, and 11 colleges. The area includes many low-income, high-density communities and an inadequate public transportation system.

Since its inception in August, 1966, the San Gabriel Valley Mental Health Service has emphasized the preventive functions of the community mental health center: mental health consultation, professional and lay education, and community involvement. At the same time, the service has maintained an outpatient treatment service offering individual, group, conjoint, and family therapy. The original 21-position module standard for the Department of Mental Health Regional Services, proposing to serve that 1,500,000 residents of the San Gabriel Valley, consisted of 15 professionals: four psychiatrists, one psychologist, three nurses, four psychiatric social workers, one community services coordinator, one vocational rehabilitation counselor, and one medical case worker. The present multidiscipline staff consists of two full-time psychiatrists (including the regional chief), two part-time psychiatrists, one psychologist, five psychiatric social workers, three nurses, two medical case workers, one vocational rehabilitation counselor, one recreational therapist, one community services coordinator, and 10 clerical positions.

Recently, California mental health legislation has added to the San Gabriel Service the responsibility for implementing the Lanterman-Petris-Short Act. The Act broadens the scope of direct service to include emergency teams that provide personnel for screening patients for involuntary and voluntary admissions to hospitals in the public sector. These teams also provide services such as crisis intervention therapy in the clinic, home visits when indicated, and coordination with local police departments.

Our future plans include an additional 21 position module and a day-night treatment unit. When staffing is complete, nursing will have a total of 12 professional positions and four psychiatric technician positions.

During my experience with the agency, various disciplines were assigned major consultation responsibility: psychiatrists would provide consultation to non-psychiatric physicians and the clergy; psychologists to schools, law-enforcement and correctional agencies; psychiatric social workers to welfare agencies; and nurses to nursing agencies and groups in the catchment area. Although there were and are no hard and fast rules regarding these dividing lines, the major responsibility for responding to requests for consultation was according to discipline, educational preparation, and experience. The rationale for assigning responsibility in this manner was based primarily on staff interest in the specified areas. Such a division of labor has given rise to interesting observations and it is my intention in this paper to contrast functioning as a nurse mental health consultant with one's own discipline, as opposed to mental health consultation with other disciplines.

The two main consultee groups providing the material this experience is based on are community nursing groups and teaching and ancillary staff of Headstart programs—dietitians, community aides, social workers, and so on. When consulting with other disciplines, the consultant has to learn new systems and roles as well as the skills used by the consultee. Such occurrences as consultee resistance, or the tendency to slip into other and more familiar roles, are difficulties faced by any consultant, but the ease with which one slips into the role of supervisor, for example, is of less concern when disciplines are different; presumably, the reduced concern is due to a lack of knowledge in the consultee's field. This lack of knowledge, however, places a responsibility on the consultant to learn the system the agency exists in, its program and philosophy, as well as a refreshing of one's memory with regard to specifics of the client population—in other words, with respect to the Headstart program, child behavior, characteristics of various age groups, and so on.

CONCEPTS OF MENTAL HEALTH CONSULTATION

A sound foundation in and knowledge of behavior are essential in doing mental health consultation. "Well-trained psychotherapists learn important aspects of mental health consultation fairly easily. They are able to use their understanding of unconcious processes and their interpersonal sensitivities and skills in the assessment of the inner-meaning of the behavior and communications of the consultee in fostering the consultation relationship."[9]

Frequently, a consultant will find that a group initially designated for consultation will, on closer examination, be found in need of mental health education. In my work with numerous nursing groups, I have found that they are required to deal more and more with a mental patient population they are unfamiliar with and that they lack basic knowledge regarding treatment modalities, drugs, preventive concepts, and so on. Using the consultation process (usually either the client or consultee-centered model), gaps in the consultees' factual knowledge become apparent to the consultant. The consultant then needs to recognize a possible need for a shift in focus, and must be able to adopt a new stance and schedule a conference with administration to present impressions and recommendations. It is important to be willing—and flexible enough—to provide material as indicated instead of remaining rigidly in an original consultation model. In other words, the consultant must have flexibility as well as knowledge of what model is being used at all times.

Part of my experience of broadening mental health education to a nontraditional group of community caretakers, has been as a consultant to leaders of Camp Fire Girls. Mental health education for this group has taken the form of providing information on the characteristics of girls aged seven through 17 but the major emphasis has been on principles of group dynamics and how to deal with groups. As an example, how do leaders deal with the shy, the bossy, or the indifferent girl? The community caretakers in this instance were responsible individuals at times for a large segment of the "well" population. A continuing responsibility of mental health educators is to keep the lay and professional publics informed about community mental health centers, new mental health legislation, and the like and, in our Service, it has been of primary importance to respond to requests from PTA's, service clubs and professional groups, for speakers.

CONSULTANT-CONSULTEE RELATIONSHIPS: DIFFERENT BACKGROUNDS

The definition of mental health consultation I am most familiar with is an egalitarian process in which the consultant and consultee are both competent professionals, but in different fields. Here, it is assumed that the consultant has more knowledge and expertise in an area other than that of the consultee. But, what if the consultant has more knowledge and expertise in the *same* area as the consultee? What are the advantages, if any, of this type of relationship? What are the complications that may develop when this particular relationship exists?

If the consultant has expertise in the same area as the consultee, the consultation is a departure from the traditional model. The advantages become immediately apparent. In my experience, community nursing agencies (health departments, visiting nurse associations, general hospital staffs) and their systems were familiar to me. Although I had never worked in some of these agencies, my experience as both a basic and graduate student, in addition to actual employment, provided first-hand knowledge of the systems and their functioning. Likewise, the roles, functions, and job specifications of the consultees were well known to me. Considering these two factors—knowledge of a system one enters into as a consultant, and some understanding of the roles and functions of consultees—as essential to effective consultation, previously acquired knowledge in these areas would appear to be primarily beneficial.

In my work with nursing groups, however, there appeared to be two significant occurrences: (1) many of the nursing agencies would rigidly restrict the consultant's time for consultation, restrict the number of visits per month, and manifest persistent ambivalence; (2) the temptation for the consultant to slip into the role of supervisor was ever present. It is well known by anyone who functions as a consultant that ambivalence, scheduling problems, and so on represent typical resistances. These often are not very different from the resistances of patients undergoing psychotherapy. I am indebted to Dr. Walter E. Brackelmanns and the Advanced Mental Health Consultation and Education Professional Study Group at the Center for Training in Community Psychiatry, Los Angeles, for bringing out the principle that, "When an organization does something to the consultant which, at first glance, appears to inhibit or constrict his effectiveness, the first way a consultant should attempt to view this is to consider the ways in which the system is protecting itself and setting up a relationship which will allow it to use the consultant in the most effective way under the complicated existing circumstances."[10] In other words, the "complicated existing circumstances" in my experience consisted of functioning as a consultant both knowledgeable in the consultee's field and possessing expertise in the field of mental health. The need for the system to protect itself in such circumstances is related to and closely tied in with my second observation, and that is the ease with which one can slip (albeit unintentionally), from the role of consultant into the role of supervisor. This departure from the role of consultant is always a hazard for any consultant, but in my experience, the likelihood appears higher when consultant and consultee are in the same discipline.

Such experience points out the necessity for adequate preparation and training in the consultation role and the development of one's own consultation model. The model I usually operate with is client-centered or consultee-centered as described by Caplan.[11] The finer nuances of the process of consultation come with experience, and, consequently, the best route becomes clearer to the consultee's goal of growth and independence. Without such preparation and training (which I received at the Center for Training in Community Psychiatry, mentioned above), the tendency is to fall back on and use well known, old skills one is comfortable with. One of these more familiar skills may be supervision in an agency where consultant and consultee are of the same discipline. Such departure into another role is particularly true when the consultant has the ability to evaluate the actual nursing performance of the consultee. As I see it, evaluation of performance is not the function of the consultant and, should the consultant depart from this role and become a "supervisor," the destructiveness of such a maneuver to the agency is obvious; to function effectively, the consultant must allow the consultee freedom of choice in deciding on a course of action and must have no stake in the consultee's performance. These elements are clearly and rightfully present in the supervisor-supervisee relationship but would eventually destroy the consultant-consultee relationship.

What effect does the appearance of the nurse consultant in a nursing agency have on the administrator, director, or supervisor of such an agency? I believe that a nurse consultant can pose a real threat to nurses in administrative positions in these agencies. Here again, a consultant is frequently very threatening to individuals in administrative positions in recipient agencies. In my experience, however, where the consultant was of the same discipline, the threat (as demonstrated by rigid limit-setting), appeared greater by virtue of the fact that often the consultant was educationally better-prepared in nursing generally and, if not having expertise, at least was skillful in (or knowledgeable about) the functions of the nurse consultees. Under these circumstances, to make oneself a valuable person to agencies requires skill and experience.

In conclusion, it is my feeling that the core of mental health consultation and education for nursing or any other discipline lies in adequate preparation and training. Consultation is not direction, supervision, or teaching but—there are components of each in the consultant-consultee relationship. The responsibility for maintaining performance in a role that is fraught with the difficulties already mentioned requires a solid foundation of experience and formalized training. Nurses without such preparation cannot readily assume this role with respect to their assistance to community caretakers.

REFERENCES

1. U.S. Department of Health, Education and Welfare. Health, Education and Welfare Trends, Part 1, National Trends, 1964 Edition. Washington, D.C., U.S. Department of Health, Education and Welfare, 1964, p. xi.
2. California Department of Mental Hygiene. Pattern of Progress. Sacramento, Calif., State Printing Office, 1962, p. 31.
3. Los Angeles County Department of Mental Health. Plan For Mental Health Services Fiscal Year 1970-71. Los Angeles, California, Los Angeles County Department of Mental Health, 1969. p. 3.
4. Los Angeles County Department of Mental Health, Evaluation and Research Division. Patient and Service Statistics January, 1968, Report No. 5. Los Angeles, California, Los Angeles County Department of Mental Health, 1968, p. 17.

5. Personal communication with Evaluation and Research Division, Los Angeles County Department of Mental Health.
6. Churchill, J. An issue: Nurses and psychotherapy. Perspect. Psychiat. Care, 5:160-162, 1967.
7. De Paul, A.V. The Nurse as a Central Figure in a Mental Health Center. Perspect. Psychiat. Care, 6:17-24, 1968.
8. Lessler, K., Bridges, J. The Psychiatric Nurse in a Mental Health Clinic. Ment. Hyg., 49:324-330, 1965.
9. Caplan, G. Problems of Training In Mental Health Consultation In Concepts of Community Psychiatry, framework for training. S.E. Goldston, ed. Washington, D.C., ([Public Health Service Publication 1319]; National Institute of Mental Health.) 1965, p. 103.
10. Brackelmanns, W. E., Unpublished material. Center for Training in Community Psychiatry, Los Angeles, California.
11. Caplan, G. Principles of Preventive Psychiatry. New York, Basic Books, Inc., 1964, p. 214-227.

ADDITIONAL REFERENCES

Brickman, H. R. Community mental health—means or end?
Psychiatric Digest, 28:43-50, 1967.
Brickman, H. R. The new mental health system.
Calif. Med., 109:403-408, 1968.

DISCUSSION

Question:

The Lanterman-Petris-Short Act drastically changed mental health services in California. What were the effects of this law on patients?

Miss Martois:

Primarily, the law was designed to guarantee the civil rights of patients. For example, the right to obtain a driver's license, the right to vote, a right to trial, and so on. In addition, the law took away the right of the hospital to give electric shock treatment without the patient's consent and guaranteed that all signs would be posted in English and Spanish. However, some patients were bewildered by the concrete changes, and some could not accept the underlying philosophy. Patients now had to be screened for both voluntary and involuntary admissions to the state hospital in their local neighborhood. It has been a hardship on patients by and large; people who had been in the state hospital were used to just going there and being admitted. They travel there, which is about 25-30 miles from our office, and are told, "You cannot be admitted. You must be screened by the regional service first." Then they have to drive the 25 or 30 miles back. We screen them and, in general, we don't recommend admission for them; they're not accustomed to this kind of procedure. So, the community people are somewhat distressed by it, particularly the ex-patient population who are again requesting service, and they don't quite understand how it works.

In an attempt to localize services, the law provided for emergency services in the county. In fact, the state of California "wants out" of the mental health "business" and wants to turn it over to the counties entirely. The plan is to regionalize the state hospitals and divide them up among the counties. The counties will eventually administer the facility.

Although no one questioned the civil rights part of the law, there was a great deal of resistance to the other part because counties were not ready for it; there was very little planning, and what planning there was not compatible with the interests of the patients and the programs already in existence. Eventually we will operate a service seven days a week, 24 hours a day for emergencies and for the admission and screening of patients. At the present time, we are only able to operate five days a week from 8:00 A.M. to 3:00 P.M. The state or county hospital serve as a back-up for the remainder of the day which, at this time, is confusing to patients and their families.

Question:

What is your relationship to the state hospital?

Miss Martois:

When they rearranged the hospitals in the county, all hospitals were designated either "primary" or "back-up" hospitals. In our catchment area, our first hospital is County General Hospital, which has a 200-bed psychiatric unit. Our second hospital (that is our back-up hospital), is a 1,000-bed metropolitan state hospital. We are not doing consultation with the state hospital, but we do work closely as liaison agents with them in terms of patients who are admitted and discharged from the hospital. We have an equally active role with the county hospital because most of our patients go there first. The Lanterman-Petris-Short Act forced us into this kind of service, which we were not doing adequately before.

Question:

How much have the changes in the law affected your role in terms of your consultation services to the community?

Miss Martois:

The changes in the law have affected my role in that the amount of consultation is limited. The funding is for direct service; therefore, direct service holds the highest priority. The nurse cares for the emergencies, screens patients, goes out with the police; these activities are taken care of first and then consultation and community education follow in whatever time there is left. For example, two weeks ago we spent two whole days on emergency service call walk-in clinics, hundreds of police calls, and that kind of thing. In addition, since I am part of the administrative staff, I lead one therapy group, carry five individual patients, and supervise the nurses working with me. I have very little time for consultation, which is where the pay-off is. It's most unfortunate for there have been several groups in need of consultation: the public health nurses from a county health department and three diferent visiting nurse association groups; hospital nursing staffs; industrial nurses and some school nurses; and Headstart personnel.

Question:
As consultants, what was your entree into the various agencies? Was it a mandate?

Miss Martois:
The entree part of consultation takes the most finesse and the most skill. Consultation cannot be mandated. We began the consultation service by going out and introducing ourselves to the personnel of the various agencies in the catchment area—it's about 30 miles east and west and about 18 miles north and south—a large area to cover! We initiated contacts with the welfare, health and probation departments, and discussed and offered our services to them. Some agencies responded well and some did not. Some health department supervisors ordered their supervisees to participate; others asked their staff to volunteer for this kind of program.

We are beginning to operate a joint program with the visiting nurses in two or three districts. They carry the bulk of these patients and we offer them consultation. There are three visiting nurse agencies in my catchment area; I've had ongoing consultation programs in all of them and these nurses are really struggling with a lack of knowledge about current treatment modalities. They are frightened by patients; they dislike going into the homes and they need all the support they can get.

Comment:
In my state, we are running into the geriatric patient problem. Our nursing staff has been innovative in that we have been adamant in making the family the focus of attention, using visits and family therapy skills in this area. This shift in the patient population to the community goes hand in hand with new legislation that keeps people out of the hospital. Family members return home from distant states, having been discharged from a state hospital after some 20 to 30 years. They arrive at the son or daughter's home and create new problems. Many are still police and neighborhood nuisances and they cannot be "put away" again. It

has become very difficult to commit or involuntarily hospitalize an individual in my state.

Comment:

We have to look at the kind of available resources in a community and not push professional resources but organization resources—I mean the people in the community. We have a large geriatric program, the Senior Citizens Group. One of the problems is the geriatric patient: what to do with these isolated, alienated, or paranoid geriatric people who live alone? We are trying to get our mobile geriatric people who are actively involved in the senior citizens group to, somehow or other, connect with the immobile geriatric people in the home. Right now, we are doing it on a volunteer basis; for example, we had one woman, about 80 years old, referred to us. She was living in a basement apartment, and was becoming increasingly more paranoid. Her family lived in another state. Neighbors were afraid to approach her because she was almost psychotic and in her paranoia wouldn't let anyone in. One would think that she should be hospitalized. If you bring her into the center, what are you going to do with her? Are you going to transfer her out to the state hospital? Well, rather than do that, our mobile treatment team, a nurse and a mental health assistant, and a volunteer from the senior citizens geriatric program went in and started working with her to see if they could support her in the home situation. The geriatric volunteer, with support, will continue to visit when needed.

Comment:

As long as we keep focusing on the professional and as long as psychiatry focuses on the process of excluding problems by taking patients out of their community and putting them either in a community mental health center, (which is another community), or a state hospital, there just aren't going to be enough facilities and there aren't enough professionals. I think that what we have to do is learn how to take care of people in the communities and use the resources available within the communities they live in.

Question:

Is the graduate degree necessary for nursing practice in community mental health?

Miss Martois:

It may not be necessary for nurses in any other field except education and community mental health, but in our area we work with professionals who have earned master's and doctoral degrees. You have to have the knowledge, the skills, and the self-confidence to collaborate as a team member.

Comment:

What you're saying is great but a nurse with a master's degree won't even come to our state. We have managed to work together with a multidiscipline team who have the advanced degrees. We have learned through hard work, experience, and continuing education. We have acquired the self-confidence and the status necessary to collaborate effectively.

A Role for Nursing in a Community Drug Addiction Program

JUDITH B. PROCTOR, R.N.

To understand the pressing need for a nursing role in the treatment of drug addiction, it may be helpful to emphasize the scope of the illness. The 1967 Task Force Report on Narcotics and Drug Abuse, revealed that: "As of December, 1965, the Federal Bureau of Narcotics reported . . . 57,199 active addicts in the United States.* The Report also pointed out: "Federal Bureau of Narcotics summaries have been criticized . . . as underreporting offenders," and "National estimates by others generally reflect larger figures than reported by FBN (Federal Bureau of Narcotics). These range up to 200,000 active addicts." The Report admits that "there is no present way to verify any of the estimates; those who claim 180,000 active opiate addicts might be correct." These conflicting statistics are evidence that true accuracy in determining the range of the drug problem is quite impossible. My feeling is that these figures are conservative since an addict only gets counted when he is arrested or seeks treatment.

Recognition of the range of the drug problem created the development of a variety of programs to meet the needs of addicts. I am a staff member in one such comprehensive program. In our program we see all drug users from age fourteen up, with the exception of "glue sniffers." There are six components of the program. One is "Daytop House," a residential treatment facility run by

*The President's Commission on Law Enforcement and Administration of Justice. *Task Force Report: Narcotics and Drug Abuse* (Washington, D.C., 1967), p. 27.

ex-addicts; its policy is total drug abstinence. A second component is the "Outpatient Clinic;" it focuses on the problems of adolescent drug abusers and uses group, family, and individual therapies. It offers day status programs supplying short-term goals to its patients from which they obtain a sense of personal worth. "NARCO, Inc." is a third component; it is a storefront run by ex-addicts, located in the black ghetto of the community, and thus easily accessible to the addicts. The "Educational and Preventive" component is involved with the schools and community organizations; it provides training for those teaching drug education. The fifth component, the "Research Unit," is attempting to isolate and study factors that contribute to the successful treatment of addiction. The sixth component, the "Methadone Maintenance Unit," treats only opiate-addicted adults with the use of medication and therapy. I will focus on "Methadone Maintenance" since I have been most intimately involved in the development of the nursing role in this area.

Perhaps I can elaborate first on the reasons Methadone is most useful. It is a synthetic opiate which has certain characteristics which enable an opiate-addicted individual to function as if he were "clean;" by that I mean free from drugs. When used daily in a maintenance dose of 70 to 125 milligrams, Methadone will stop drug craving without creating a euphoric feeling. It can be taken orally with any flavored drink or water; its action is sustained over a 24-hour period, and it is relatively inexpensive. Perhaps its most useful side effect is the blockading of heroin. A person maintained on an appropriate dose of Methadone will not feel the effects of heroin, opium, or its derivatives.

THE BEGINNING OF OUR PROGRAM

Before we began our program two years ago, we were warned (by others who had used Methadone) against housing our patients in a psychiatric setting. They felt that addicts did not view their problem as psychiatric, and that any inference to the contrary would be highly resented and might result in hostile behavior on the addicts' part. We evaluated a number of facilities, but a mental health center offered the only space available so we contracted for three, 24-hour beds on a psychiatric research division in that center.

On admission, our patients immediately seemed to feel a need to do two things: first, they wanted to prove that they were not like other patients, and this was consistent with the warning we had received; second, they attempted to pit the drug unit staff against the regular division staff. There were only enough drug-involved staff to cover one shift of duty from 7:30 A.M. to 4:00 P.M. The hostility between staff members was felt most acutely on the evening and night shifts. During the day, the channels for communication were available, but the lack of drug-involved staff made communication virtually impossible on the other shifts. Not only was insufficient staff coverage a problem, but contracting for only three beds on a 24-hour basis cut down the number of admissions we were able to accept at any one time.

The psychiatric structure was made up of three teams, each with its own resident and nursing staff; each 24-hour patient was assigned to one of these teams. The philosophy of treatment was inconsistent because the floor teams' orientations were primarily intrapsychic while the drug-involved staff saw day-to-day, reality problems of greater importance. The intrapsychic approach entailed a number of months for treatment; concentrating on reality issues implied a much shorter inpatient stay. Having the addict in the hospital around the clock reduced staff's ability to work with the incidents the patient would face because he was removed from his environment.

In view of these problems, a serious assessment of the total program was made three months and eight patients after its beginning. As a result of the assessment, we tried taking patients on an ambulatory basis, that is, outpatients who came for daily medication and one group therapy session a week. We found this unsatisfactory because staff felt that they had little investment in the patients since they did not know them well; the patients felt little commitment to the program or to each other. A month later, we started a whole new induction system. We traded our three 24-hour beds for 10 day-status slots, and that now has become our primary mode of admission. Patients come in from 8:30 A.M. to 4:00 P.M., five days a week. On Saturdays and Sundays, they only come in to obtain their medication.

At the time our induction method changed and we moved to a day-status program, our treatment style also changed. The therapeutic emphasis switched from individual to group therapy. Individual therapy was offered only in cases of special need. With the formation of a 10-patient day team, it was possible for drug-involved staff to assume responsibility for the administration and treatment of the addict patients. At the same time, the drug program became the fourth on the existing unit with a homogeneous patient group.

ROLE OF THE COUNSELORS

The drug team staffing consisted of one psychiatrist, responsible for the total comprehensive program as its director; one social worker, director of the outpatient clinic; one vocational counselor primarily involved with financial assistance and employment agencies; three registered nurses, including myself; and one rehabilitation counselor. The rehabilitation counselor is an ex-addict who has come through our Methadone program; he may or may not be maintained currently on Methadone. At present, all of the counselors happen to be Methadone-maintained. The source for the rehabilitation counselor is the patient population of the program; men I worked with originally as patients are now staff members. A patient is considered for one of these positions if he has shown individual motivation for change as evidenced by steady employment, abstinence from drugs, and positive changes in his life style.

In the nursing staff, the combination of rehabilitation counselors and professional nurses gives us a special working style. Our counselors come from a black ghetto where they have led a drug life for many years. The nurses' lives are quite different from the counselors and the patients. The major contributions of the counselors lie in their ability to work directly with patients and to advise the professional medical staff on the basis of their past experience. In contrast, the professional nurse offers an academic understanding of the problems of drug abuse, and psychiatric knowledge and experience. The combination of these assets has provided the nursing backbone to this program. Both the counselors and the nurses share a commitment to patient care; their success in treatment is based on a collaborative effort; in other words, neither has as much to offer alone. The process of working out inter-staff differences—culturally, racially, socially, and so on—has enabled each staff member to give better patient care. One method we employed to understand some of the cross-cultural differences was a brief workshop (eight sessions) with readings and discussions on black and white cultures. As a result of our sharing, the counselor has a better understanding of the theory behind addiction as an illness, and the nurse has a better appreciation of the life problems of her patient.

The nursing staffs' role expanded markedly at this point. Out of necessity, nursing staff was largely responsible for therapy groups in the day-status program, and this brought a certain flavor to the group because of the makeup of nursing staff. In line with the philosophy of the program, the groups were designed to concentrate on reality issues. Besides working with everyday problems, we emphasized patient responsibility. It was our feeling that allowing patients to assume responsibility for their own treatment and the treatment of others would increase their sense of self-worth and their ability to deal with the outside world. Each patient was seen as having responsiblity for himself, other patients, and the total program.

PATIENT INVOLVEMENT

Patients are very involved in the running of the program and this is demonstrated in a variety of ways. For example, when patients are on day-status, they deal as a group with any infractions of the rules that might have been incurred by their fellow members. Thus, patients who come in late or miss a day or have "dirty" urines (urines revealing use of drugs), are confronted *by the group*. They also have an advisory board made up of four patients and four staff members. The patients' representatives are elected from the evening therapy groups and are concerned with infractions of the rules or patients who are not doing well with the program in general. In addition to the advisory board, there are monthly meetings of all patients in the program to discuss the program as a whole and to consider changes that might be warranted.

Although philosophically it was the consensus of the staff that increased patient responsibility would be beneficial, it was difficult in practice to relinquish to patients control of certain aspects of treatment. Discharge from day-status, expulsion from the program, probation within the program, and other special considerations were determined by the patients for one another. The primary reason the staff experienced difficulty in relinquishing such control seemed to be a low tolerance for patient errors and the slower patient process for solving problems. Since control rested with the patient group, it became staffs' responsiblity to communicate to that group in a meaningful way their perceptions about an individual's functioning. For this process to operate successfully the development of mutual respect between staff and patients is essential. That respect is predicated on the fact that patients and staff share a mutual goal: helping drug-addicted persons to lead a more useful life for themselves and society. Each member of the group, staff and patient, has something special to contribute to the obtaining of that goal.

As it has evolved now, the Day Program averages six to ten weeks. Patients are involved in groups twice daily and spend the rest of their time in working on problems in the vocational and recreational areas. Once a patient is discharged from day-status (and this does not occur until he obtains a job), he is required to return daily for his medication, and once a week in the evening for group therapy. Patients remain in the evening groups for at least six months, and to leave after that specified time, need the vote of the other patients in their group. Urines are collected twice weekly on each patient and checked for narcotics, quinine, cocaine, and amphetamines.

SUMMARY REMARKS

We have found that this kind of day patient induction enables us to treat more patients and, at the same time, we can be involved in the life of each patient. Had we continued the program on the 24-hour model, we would have been able—to this date—to treat only 24 patients. As of October 1969, with the day program, we had treated 71. In contrast to the low rentention rates generally found in addiction treatment programs, we had retained 79 percent of our patients. In addition, having day patients return home every evening to cope with life in the streets, and with their family problems has made these areas accessible as issues in the therapy groups, thus facilitating an intimate involvement that did not occur when patients were hospitalized 24 hours a day.

I would like to highlight what I view as important considerations nursing personnel need to assess in relation to working in a community drug addiction program. First is an understanding of the socioeconomic subculture from which the patients come. Such understanding has occurred in our program through the working relationships of nurses and rehabilitation counselors. Second is the ability of staff members to relinquish traditional controls in patient treatment. In our program this was facilitated by establishing peer group control. And third is increasing staff tolerance of a slower moving process with the possibility of patient errors. That is a more difficult problem to solve and is resolved only when mutual respect exists between staff and patients.

Both the program and the nursing role in the program have not reached the ideal stage. There is a continuous need for work in all the areas I have isolated and talked about. What is important ultimately is defining the areas and working to resolve them.

DISCUSSION

Question:

What special training did you have to prepare you to work in the drug addiction program?

Mrs. Proctor:

The community mental health program director wanted to hire a nurse (although he did not envision how nursing would operate in the program). I subsequently was hired and worked in the psychiatric unit for six months until the project was funded. During this phase, I read all the available materials on drug addiction and relevant problems.

I started working with admitted drug addicts one at a time and thus my on-the-job training began. As I mentioned in my paper, almost all the nurses were white and almost all the patients and counselors were black. The most valuable preparation was a brief workshop. It was not the usual sensitivity training, but a cross-cultural sharing, a comparing of differences. For example, we shared different expectations different kinds of responses to certain charged words and ideas. The workshop also included recommended reading materials and discussions on black and white culture. The program ran each week for eight, two-hour sessions and it is repeated periodically. This kind of learning experience is absolutely essential, not only to provide better service to patients, but to foster the individual's personal growth as a human being.

Question:

What method do you use to select your counselors?

Mrs. Proctor:

We hire only ex-addicts who have been through our program. It is difficult to describe, but if the ex-addict is employed for a number of months and has changed his pattern of living, he becomes an eligible candidate. Some have been hard-core addicts from five to fifteen years. Their lives have been a continuous hustle to obtain money for drugs.

Question:

Would you describe the group, its goals, and how you are involved?

Mrs. Proctor:

It is a "confrontation" group rather than a formal therapy group. The group demands that each member give up the use of drugs, give up hustling, seek employment, go to work, and try to find different life satisfactions.

I have a responsibility to share what I feel is going on with an individual before the group makes a decision, and that demands a special kind of sharing, trusting relationship between staff and patient which infiltrates all facets of the program. For example, there is a rigid screening process run by the counselors; they will admit an addict to the program only if they feel he is seriously interested in changing his life style.

Question:

We're running into problems in our city with the availability of Methadone. It can be purchased for $2 whereas the cost of the heroin habit runs $50 to $100 daily. How have you managed *not* to become a Methadone-maintenance city?

Mrs. Proctor:

We ran into that problem in the beginning, but it stopped when the control of the basic program was turned over to the individual members; that is, the way the program is run and the value of the program became their job and responsibility. The members know that the success of the program is directly linked to how accessible Methadone is to people outside the program, how the community feels about the program, how well the members respect the program, and how the advisory council deals with infractions.

The advisory council is basically a patient-run group that is very strict and deals effectively with infractions of rules. It's very difficult to play any kind of a game with a staff member who is personally familiar with the same kind of game. There are four patient representatives to two staff representatives on the council; the patients are members of evening therapy groups. Discharged day-status patients return weekly to the evening groups.

Question:

How does the community accept these people when they go back? What method or means do you have to gain community support?

Mrs. Proctor:

We have spent much time and energy working with member "rites of passage" back into the community. Our primary ability to reach the community is through the vocational rehabilitation worker. Having worked in the community all his life, he has many community links. He personally endorses our members. He helps them obtain employment where there is opportunity for progressive raises in salary and status, and where the ex-addict is valued. Many of our ex-addicts have become neighborhood and community workers. They are interested and motivated to work in the community, helping others in a variety of programs.

Another crucial facet of community support is the result of our collaboration with the police and penal systems. We interpret our philosophy and practice to them, keep them informed of our progress, and consult with them on problems. In turn, they do not interfere with the work of the program. For example, the police are aware that if they arrest a client-member from our hospital, the community people would never seek out the kind of services we provide.

Question:

Do you think you are getting to some of the basic problems these people have rather than just keeping them off drugs and out of jail?

Mrs. Proctor:

Internally, many of the problems still exist; but the external behavior has been modified in a way that makes the client's life more rewarding.

Comment:

Your paper and the discussion that followed clearly point out how one nurse carved out a critical role and expanded it as the changing needs of clients and community became visible. We need to further communicate what we've discovered in a way that makes sense to other professionals. Where I'm working, most of the professionals were not going out into the homes in the neighborhood—were not responding immediately to the needs of the community. Nurses began to operate when and where the problem existed, on a 24-hour period. If the client needs us in the home for four hours to help him organize himself during a crisis, we can get the kids taken care of; or if he needs us to go to court and to help him fight the court system, or if someone needs help in getting bailed out of jail, or if one of our workers needs to be picked up in prison, I'm going to *do* or get someone else out to help *do*, but I am going to do something that I feel is useful. I have something to give to people in the community. In one crisis situation, we had to get three families living on one street to meet in someone's living room. Working when and where the problem is happening means that if someone is trying to shoot someone next door, it is foolhardy to ask them to come in for an appointment.

In the beginning there were only one or two nurses moving out into the community; then we took a paraprofessional along with us. As we gained some skill and experience, additional nurses and paraprofessionals were hired. In this way, we increased all our potentials and responses to crises calls were rotated among individuals. Furthermore, when I started groups, I included the paraprofessional from the beginning. His on-the-job training enabled him to develop the necessary skills to prepare him for working alone.

Comment:

For too long nurses have allowed other people to define nursing roles instead of deciding for ourselves what we can and should do. Nursing prepares us to be flexible to work almost anyplace—in the home, in an office, even on a street corner. I think this is unique to nursing; it should be defined as practice, enhanced, and valued, not just by us, and not just by patients, but by the health community.

I can go into a home and reach out and build a relationship with the client, and this enables us to learn from each other. The patient has to determine the alternatives to solve his problems.

Comment:

The recurrent question is, "How can we explain to other professionals what we do and how we do it?" Perhaps this is unimportant and unnecessary. All we have to do is demonstrate that we're doing it and other disciplines who want nothing to do with crisis intervention turn over to nursing all crisis intervention. We must accept this until others are ready to assist. What we should be concerned about is that we are financially rewarded for these services.

ORGANIZATIONAL STRUCTURE AND ADMINISTRATIVE PRACTICE

During the past decade, the Federal government mandated a comprehensive plan of health service to meet the health needs of communities. Increased mental health facilities are one component of this plan. The legislation was intended to improve the nature and delivery of such mental health services to the residents of the local communities.

As funds are made available to communities for the establishment of new patterns of service, vying is intense between agencies for control of funds. In addition, mental health agencies want to promulgate their ideology and practices thus becoming a part of the overall process. Trends indicate that there is an urgent need for the formation of coalitions. The administrative practices of mental health organizations must be viewed and understood in the context of their relationships to external systems.

Community mental health organizational patterns are characterized by a decentralization of structure which, together with changing policies, purports to delegate authority to various points of reference. This shift in power, from a stable system to a new and often unstable one, requires a change in roles and values. Role relationships emerge and influence the way in which mental health resources and services are made available.

Nursing is one group in the mental health organization. Historically, nurses have carried out activities in the community that make entry less problematic, and this precedent may also serve to enhance their negotiating powers with community residents. However, nurses continue their struggle to attain status and power in the professional arena and often feel powerless to affect change. Conferees pointed to nursing education and clinical experiences which promote a holistic orientation to patient care and also expouse interagency and interdisciplinary collaboration as a basis for enhancing nursing's potential as a change agent.

Like other mental health professionals, nurses deplore the regulatory structure and administrative policies that block the accessibility and availability of help to those who need it.

Speakers viewed the sources of power and the efficacy of certain structures and noted attempts on the part of nurses to mobilize themselves and others in addressing crucial organizational models. The speakers focused attention on the fact that nurses frequently operated in the medical-model framework despite their sociocultural orientation. As a result of this experience many nurses are sensitized to the importance of eliciting and supporting community participation in establishing program priorities and meaningful structures. In striving to reach this objective, community mental health nurses generate diverse expectations, anxieties, resistances, and disappointments among agency personnel, clients, community factions, and themselves. It is evident that nurses along with others are beginning to appreciate the impact of structure on practice and the need to become more sophisticated in assessing systems and their constraints.

Organizational Structure and Administrative Practice as they Affect the Nurse's Role

NORMAN MORSE, R.N., M.A.

The community health movement requires new and innovative methods, techniques, and practices to achieve its stated goals. To reach these goals, the Maimonides Community Mental Health Center, Brooklyn, New York has devised an innovative system for the delivery of its services. This paper will include a general overview of the organizational structure of the Maimonides Community Mental Health Center (as of January, 1969), an analysis of the administrative practices, and how these two elements combine to affect the role of the nurse in this type of setting. Although there are many factors that have implications for nursing, I will place greatest emphasis on the concepts of power and authority.

The Maimonides Community Mental Health Center (hereafter MCMHC) is a part of the Maimonides Medical Center. The present operation of the MCMHC began in 1961 as the Department of Psychiatry. Initially, the department provided only outpatient services, adding liaison services and a community development program as it grew. A separate structure on the Medical Center grounds was completed early in 1968 and all five mandated elements of service were in partial operation by June of that year. Thus it has been only in the past year and a half that a full range of services has been offered—a rather rapid development.

The catchment area served by the MCMHC includes more than 100,000 people and encompasses several natural communities. The boundaries of the catchment area are those of four adjacent New York City Health Districts, with the MCMHC situated approximately in the center of these districts. The population is predominantly a lower socioeconomic group. The cultural communities are demonstrating some changes but consist mostly of the following: large Jewish, Scandinavian, and Italian groups, a rapidly increasing Puerto Rican group, and a small but growing black community.

It is with this background and in this community setting that the organizational structure I am going to outline was instituted in the fall of 1967. It was also at this time that the MCMHC enlarged its staff by about two-thirds to its present size of approximately 150 members. The staff includes: psychiatrists, psychiatric social workers, group workers, community organization workers, psychologist, psychiatric nurse clinicians (with masters' degrees), staff nurses, a social scientist, educational psychologists, remedial teachers, a vocational counsellor, art and dance therapists, research staff, indigenous mental health workers, and housekeeping, dietary, and clerical personnel.

The staff provides not only the five essential services of its mandate (outpatient, inpatient, partial hospitalization, 24-hour emergency services, and community education and consultation programs), but other services as well. Some examples include the liaison team, which provides services to the Medical Center; child psychiatry; reading rehabilitation services; mental retardation consultation and outpatient services; and the research unit, which has been conducting dream research and studies on extrasensory perception. Although other community mental health centers provide these and additional services, each center has its own special structure to facilitate delivery of these services.

ORGANIZATIONAL STRUCTURE

The organizational structure of the MCMHC may be considered in four general areas: administrative, disciplinary, service, and coordinating functions. The ultimate responsibility for the functioning of the Center falls to the three directors, whom I have labeled the administrative group (Table 1, A).

The disciplinary group is represented by the directors of all staff groupings both in and outside the agency (Table 1, B). Each of these staff groups are the same as those usually encountered in agencies where each disciplinary group has a separate identity from that of the agency. A nurse, for example, is a member of the nursing service that functions in a particular agency. The Community Leaders' Group is composed of the leaders of various community organizations, such as the parent-teacher associations, block associations, religious groups, and so on. The Mental Health Assistants Group is represented primarily by the director of nursing, but also may be represented by the director of a service group.

The service groups are each represented by the directors of those units, with the exception of the General Service Groups (Table 1, C). The General Service

Table 1.

MAIMONIDES COMMUNITY MENTAL HEALTH CENTER
ORGANIZATIONAL STRUCTURE AS OF JANUARY, 1969

A.   ADMINISTRATIVE GROUP

Director (Psychiatrist)
Associate Director for Clinical Services (Psychiatrist)
Associate Director of Community Services, Administrator (Social Worker)

B.   DISCIPLINARY GROUP

Director of Community Leaders' Group
      "   " Community Organization Services
      "   " Dietary Services
      "   " Group Work Services
      "   " Housekeeping Services
      "   " Nursing Services
      "   for Psychiatrists' Group (Associate Director for Clinical Services)
      "   of Psychological Services
      "   " Social Work Services
      "   " Volunteers (Group Worker)
Mental Health Assistants Group (Director of Nursing and others)
Office Manager (for clerical services)

C.   SERVICE GROUP

Director of Child Psychiatry Services
      "   " Hospitalization Services
      "   " Learning Rehabilitation Services
      "   " Liaison Services
      "   " Mental Retardation Unit
      "   " Research Unit
General Service Group Coordinators

D.   COORDINATING COMMITTEE

Administrative Group
Disciplinary Group
Directors of Service Units
Either Coordinator from each General Service Group
One elected representative from each General Service Group and
    from the Hospitalization Unit
A second representative from the Community Leaders' Group

Group (GSG) in our organization replace the more conventional child, adolescent, and adult clinics. These groups are the basic service units of the Center, and each of the four groups is assigned a specific geographical section of the catchment area and given the responsibility of providing and coordinating all services in that area. All Center staff are assigned originally to one of these

Table 2.

MAIMONIDES COMMUNITY MENTAL HEALTH CENTER
ORGANIZATIONAL STRUCTURE

A.   GENERAL SERVICE GROUPS

   Medical Coordinator
   Administrative Coordinator
   Multidisciplinary Staff (staff nurses not in this group at present)

B.   HOSPITALIZATION UNIT

   Director
   Assistant Administrator for Hospitalization Services (non-
      psychiatric professional)
   Nurse Coordinator (psychiatric nurse clinician)
   Team Leaders (any qualified professional)
   Multidisciplinary staff

C.   RELATIONSHIPS BETWEEN COORDINATING COMMITTEE,
   TOTAL STAFF, AND THE VARIOUS FORMAL GROUPS

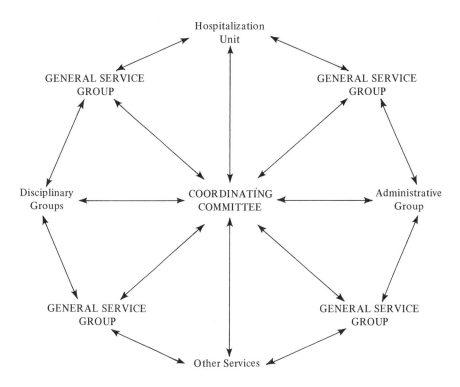

groups. The GSG is a multidisciplinary group and has only the two medical and administrative coordinator positions assigned in the group (Table 2, A). The medical coordinator is a psychiatrist assigned to assume the medicolegal responsibilities; the administrative coordinator is a nonmedical professional assigned to coordinate the clinical functions of the group. Leadership of the GSG is not assigned, but is left to each group to develop as best suits its needs. In terms of role development, this process is highly significant to the functioning of a nurse.

Each GSG has devised varying mechanisms of leadership, but each has tended to form basically similar patterns. Chairmanship of the group, for instance, is assumed on a monthly rotating basis, using all group members; case assignments are made among all professional staff on the basis of rotation and selection by the potential therapists; supervision is based on competence in particular areas. Thus a nurse is offered an unusual opportunity to develop leadership and clinical skills. As chairman for a month, a nurse would be responsible for conducting the meetings by helping to formulate agendas, determine priorities, facilitate discussions, and assist in effecting group movement. In clinical functioning, there are various concurrent opportunities available. The nurse may serve alone as primary therapist or with a cotherapist as her supervisee, her peer, or her supervisor, depending on her interests and skills and the needs of the client. This structure is particularly advantageous for the nurse clinician, who has been prepared to function both in independent and interdependent roles. Equally important in this form of multiple leadership in a group is the ability to develop not only leadership skills, but an increased sense of worth. Each nurse's contribution is valued for what it is, rather than for where the nurse is located in a hierarchical pecking order.

Another service group, the Hospitalization Unit, has its own administrative staff but does not function as a separate unit in the Center (Table 2, B and Table 1, C). Each multidisciplinary team in the Hospitalization Unit functions in conjunction with a specific GSG, as well as interdependently on the hospital unit. The nurse coordinator is responsible for the daily functioning of the unit, while the assistant administrator for hospital services assumes many of the tasks that were previously the responsibility of a head nurse. The nurse clinician functioning in the role of the nurse coordinator assumes the responsibility for consultation with and education of the hospital staff by acting as a role model, conducting informal teaching, and coordinating the milieu programs.

Staff nurses in the Hospitalization Unit also have the opportunity to broaden and strengthen their roles. In this particular service area of functioning, the team leadership positions are open to qualified professionals, and a staff nurse who may hold this position finds herself responsible for a multidisciplinary team. The development of the role of the staff nurse in the Hospitalization Unit holds the same potential as that of the nurse clinician in the GSG, though not with the same degree of independence. For example, the staff nurse functioning as a team leader has an opportunity to develop leadership skills, but within the well-defined area of the Hospitalization Unit, as opposed to the nurse clinician in a GSG, where the service functioning is very broad. Compared to more traditional units, clinical functioning in the Hospital Unit allows the staff nurse a greater degree of flexibility and increased responsiblity. She may have to develop her own means to achieve the therapeutic goals set by the team, even though she is limited to a defined area of service—the hospitalized patient.

The final area to be considered under organizational structure is that of coordination. The Coordinating Committee functions as the general policy-suggesting and decision-implementing body for the MCMHC (Table 1, D). This committee is also a decision-making group, except where the Center-wide policy decisions are proposed. These are presented at total staff meetings. Here again, how the structure fosters role development in the nurse through enhancement of a feeling of worth is apparent. It is a significant step forward when a nurse has an active and influential voice in making decisions that affect her everyday functioning. For example, nurses have been influential in developing Center policy for staffing the Hospitalization Unit. Where some personnel unfamiliar with such units were willing to accept a rigidly hierarchical staffing pattern (essentially nursing), nursing's persistent voice, both in small groups and staff meetings, opted for changes that with the help of others were eventually brought about.

In essence, the Maimonides Community Mental Health Center can be described as a well-staffed Center, providing multiple services to a large, urban community through a very special structure.

ADMINISTRATIVE PRACTICES

Before looking at administrative practices, it is necessary to mention several principles underlying the services at the MCMHC. Dr. Montague Ullman, director of the Center, lists the following principles as being those of short-term treatment: the generic worker concept, where " . . . the availability of skills and experience at many different levels among many different professionals which, when properly matched with the needs of patients, could and (does) make for a much more extended pool of manpower than would otherwise be the case;"[1] and training, which has taken the form at this point of live and group supervision.

I would add three other principles to this list: continuity of care, so that fragmentation of care between the various services and therapists is reduced to a minimum; utilization of the concepts of the therapeutic community; and the concept of participatory democracy, which should be implicit in the therapeutic community. With these principles in mind, let us now examine the administrative practices.

In order to describe the administrative practices, I will make a general analysis of the decision-making process for, as Griffiths points out, "... an understanding of the decision-making process in a particular enterprise is the key to its organizational structure."[2] In examining the decision-making process, he makes several assumptions regarding administrative functioning: (1) that administration is a generalized type of behavior found in all human organizations where its life processes are being controlled: (2) that administration is the process of directing and controlling life in a social organization; and (3) that administration's function is to develop and regulate the decision-making process.[3]

Decision-making is a dynamic process, which includes not only how the decision is made, but also how it is implemented.[4] In the present context, it is necessary to consider in which group a decision is made and in which group it is implemented. In the MCMHC, there are obviously multiple combinations to any potential decision-making process. Looking again at the organizational structure, it is apparent that a heroic attempt has been made to combine the executive and administrative functions; separating them is sometimes the greatest obstacle to smooth functioning in hierarchical structures (Table 2, C). The present structure is designed to provide a flow of the decision-making processes through, and among the various combinations of groups. An example of this flow is how applicants for staff positions are interviewed by or with various people they will be working with, and how that group participates in the decision about hiring. Let us take an applicant for a staff nurse position in the Hospitalization Unit for an example. This nurse would meet at different times with several members of the nursing staff, the hospital director, nonnursing staff, and the associate director-administrator. She would also spend a day observing the Center in full operation. On the basis of observers' opinions, plus other recommendations, the nursing staff makes a decision on whether or not to hire the applicant. From her very first contact with the Center, a nurse's importance as an individual is emphasized, thus fostering in her an increased sense of responsibility for her own role performance.

Another example of decision-making would be how a discussion on the establishment of storefront operations begins in a GSG, then moves through the coordinating committee to the general staff for a policy decision, and the moves back to the GSG for implementation or, in a case supervision conference, when the GSG recommends hospitalization for a client, the Hospitalization Unit personnel are included in the decision-making and the hospital team, in turn, incorporates the GSG therapists in the treatment program during the time the patient is hospitalized.

Two concepts essential to the examination of any organizational structure and decision-making process are those of power and authority. If one accepts the concept that power is used to control decision-making, then it becomes of primary importance in the process. "Subject to the over-all control of an institutionalized value system in the society and its subsystems (for example, MCMHC, disciplines), the central phenomenon of organization is the mobilization of *power* for the attainment of the goals of the organization."[5] Here is a key to many of the problems found in mental health center operations today—seeking power in the decision-making process in relation to values and goals that are too vague. The problem manifests itself at various times in the MCMHC in the form of an ideological struggle. The extremes of this struggle can be represented by a continuum, with the medical model at one end and some form of an ecological model at the other.

The *medical model* has a doctor-patient core. The psychiatrist diagnoses, treats, and prevents mental illness by eliminating stresses or increasing the patient's capacity to deal with stress. The medical model also ". . . views human behavior in terms of biological and medical concepts of hemostasis, health and disease. . . . Disease, in this case, is thus construed as a disordered state of bodily function, mind, or behavior, that is the result of the failure to adapt to stress."[6] Treatment and the related processes used in this model are seen only in relation to the doctor-patient relationship.

The *ecological model*, on the other hand, takes a more holistic approach. It has its basis in general systems theory and views an individual, a family, a community, and the environment as a system with subsystems in continuous, dynamic interaction.[7] In this model, intervention involves all disciplinary groups on an equal basis, utilizing modification techniques with individuals, groups, and communities. In this model, ". . . planned social and individual change (through a) democratic framework (is) accepted as fundamental."[8]

NURSING'S POSITION

Nurses command a special position in this ideological struggle by virtue of their traditional experience with the medical model. Nursing theory, however, has tended to focus its conceptual approaches to working with patients from a more holistic point of view than medicine has. Nursing, having been practiced in the medical model, although that is a compromise, is in an excellent position to identify the strengths and limitations of both extremes of the ideological struggle between the medical and ecological models. Where the medical model places the psychiatrist in priestly control of the patient, the ecological model may tend to develop the *group* into a method of social control—depending on the methods used. For example, the extreme of the ecological model might advocate using group pressure to control behavior, rather than group assistance to help an individual to develop his potential. If nurses use this knowledge in decision-making processes, they will find themselves utilizing a previously untapped source of power.

Nevertheless, nurses who begin to make use of this power may quickly find themselves losing it. The exercise of power, not having been a factor in previous situations where the nurse's voice had meaning, can be a very anxiety-provoking experience in the sense that I have described it. If a nurse begins to vocalize what may be an alternative to the ideological struggle, she has, in this setting, the unusual experience of being heard. It is at this point that she begins to exercise power and assume leadership. An example can be drawn from a clinical situation where an adolescent is exhibiting what is popularly called "school phobic behavior." A therapist operating from the medical model might want the child hospitalized or placed in a residential treatment setting; a therapist at the opposite pole may determine that the child can be benefited only if the entire family is seen together. A nurse would more probably see the adolescent as a person who is a member of a family and might suggest some combination of these two approaches. The anxiety experienced by the nurse in this newer role will, perhaps, tend to cause her to fall back on previous behavior patterns thereby reducing her anxiety. Then we see the nurse acting in the traditionally dependent position and, if not actively, then passively relinquishing her power and influence by remaining silent. I am sure any of us here can recall personal experiences when we wished we had spoken up in defense of an opinion, and yet did not for fear of being attacked, not supported, or because we did not feel ours was a justifiable view.

The implication is clear for nursing in any agency. There must be frequent communication in the nursing group that will help the group and individuals to clarify and vocalize their positions and roles, and to make a conscious and aggressive effort to support one another. If nurses do not exercise their power soon, they may find themselves replaced by the rapidly growing semiprofessional groups—physician assistants and mental health technicians.

A final concept to include in the examination of the decision-making process is that of authority. Authority is the power to make decisions that will guide the actions of others, and it includes the willingness of some to accept the power of another.[9-10] Let us look again at the organizational structure of the MCMHC and note that the basic functional units of the Center, namely the General Service Groups, locate their authority in terms of decision-making, in the group rather than in an individual. The resulting decision-making processes have sometimes been quite lengthy when opponents in the ideological struggle vie for power from a position of equal authority in the Group. The frequency of long delays in reaching group decisions seems to be, however, more a problem in administrative practice than in the organizational structure. In other words, decision-making in a group with multiple leadership and shared power is not in itself an unworkable method. However, it may be an ineffective or weak method when the group members do not continually analyze their internal processes, and when decisions must be forced through by taking a "majority vote" rather than a consensus. The persistent ideological struggles exemplify this.

Not only the method of treatment, but also values and goals are reflected in the ideological struggle, which points up poorly defined institutional values and goals by the authority—the staff. This does not, however, contradict the fact that there are goals implicit in the organization's structure and administrative practices. The origin of the conflict lies in employing conflicting administrative procedures. Sears points out that administrative function derives its purpose from the nature of the service it directs. An administrative mechanism may be formulated first and then instituted in an organization; or, the authority may first study the operating unit in terms of needs and abilities, and then tailor an administrative structure to meet the situation.[11] The first is authority-centered; the second is need-centered.[12]

Part of the present conflict at MCMHC arises from employing the first method, while trying to predict the second. In other words, an administrative structure had been designed to meet a projected need and then was put into operation with a largely new staff, instead of deriving an administrative mechanism after studying the actual staff and patient needs. In light of the structure and practice I have described, the continuation of this problem is significant not only from an administrative point of view, but also from the way the staff has handled the problem.

I have outlined previously how much freedom exists for all MCMHC staff in decision-making. The next step would seem to be that the staff would identify the problems of goals, values, and administrative practices and then formulate resolutions. The process of decision-making has demonstrated, however, that the staff frequently is unable to reach decisions by this process. The larger and more heterogeneous the group, the greater the difficulty reaching a consensus for a decision. Power seems to be the major problem; when individuals vie for power in this kind of decision-making, they frequently operate from a position of weakness. In contrast to other disciplinary groups, nurses in our agency have tended to be in a relatively strong position when they have chosen to use their power. By maintaining themselves as a primary group in their own discipline, they have been better able to clarify for themselves what the position of a nurse should be in various situations. The situation cited earlier—how nurses worked to affect opinions on hospital unit staffing—is an example of this, and again points out the necessity for nurses to constantly examine their functioning as a total group. There the potential for change is always present.

FURTHER IMPLICATIONS

Difficulty in the decision-making process represents a complexity of problems that has pertinent implications for nursing. As community mental health center practice moves from the medical model to an ecological model (and it must do this to remain viable), the power base must shift from the medical authority to a multidisciplinary group. "The medical model of psychiatry remains in use because it is socially useful to disguise the social functions of psychiatry. (It) induces us to accept the claim that the psychiatrist functions as a physician, and it induces us to prejudge his activities with the enthusiastic approval that we give to the practice of medicine."[13] As we move to the ecological model, individual responsibility for our actions increases. Community mental health nursing as such will survive only if nurses meet this challenge. Role changes necessitated by the shift from the medical model to the ecological model place a great deal of responsibility on the individual professions for a re-examination of their purposes and functions. If mental health nursing continues to divorce itself from its broad base of general nursing theory and practice, and to strive only for status by emulating the medical psychotherapists, nursing will have nothing significant at a professional level to offer community mental health programs. This is not to imply that nurses should not do psychotherapy, but it is an error to base our practice in the field of mental health on watered-down psychiatry for undergraduates or imitators on the graduate level. The actual effectiveness of any psychotherapeutic method over that of any other has yet to be supported by any really convincing evidence. If nurses will look to nursing, I think they will find a sound basis for effective therapeutic relationships through the development of nursing theory. Nursing care has become too expensive; the public will not permit us to be imitators much longer.

The Maimonides Community Mental Health Center offers very special and exciting challenges to nursing, as well as other professions. The organizational structure and administrative practices have placed the Center on one of the advanced fronts in the community mental health movement. Many of the problems I have described reflect the nature of part of the crisis in health services we face in the nation today. Nurses, along with members of other disciplines, must stop passing the buck to the physician, particularly in community mental health nursing, and they must define, communicate, and develop their own roles. Stokes has described some of the roles of psychiatric nurses at the MCMHC and adds: "We are quite convinced that other psychiatric nurses can develop the extended roles available to them within their own settings in a like manner."[14] I hope that, for the benefit of all of us, community mental health nurses throughout the country will heed this exhortation.

REFERENCES

1. Ullman, M. Overview of the evolution of the Maimonides Community Mental Health Center and the training project. The Psychiatric Nurse in Community Psychiatry. *In* Stokes, G.A., ed. The Roles of Psychiatric

Nurses in Community Mental Health Practice: A Giant Step. New York, Maimonides Medical Center—Community Mental Health Center, 1969, p. 5.

2. Griffiths, D.E. Administrative Theory. New York, Appleton-Century-Crofts, 1959, p. 80.

3. Ibid., pp. 71-74.

4. McCanny, J. Analysis of the process of decision-making. Public Admin. Rev., VII: Winter, 1947.

5. Parsons, T. Suggestions for a sociological approach to the theory of organization—II. Admin. Sci. Quart., 1:225, 1956-1957.

6. Leifer, R. In the name of mental health: social functions of psychiatry. New York, Science House, Inc., 1969, pp. 20-21.

7. Morse, N. Working with families: an ecological systems model. Clinical Nursing: Current Concepts in Selected Clinical Areas—II. Institute presented to faculty in associate degree programs in nursing, New York University, Division of Nurse Education, December, 1969, p. 2.

8. Adelson, D. A concept of comprehensive community mental health. Report of Work Conference in Psychiatric-Mental Health Graduate Education in Nursing. Baltimore, University of Maryland School of Nursing, 1967, pp. 10-13.

9. Simon, H. Administrative Behavior. New York, The Macmillan Company, 1950, p. 125.

10. Griffiths, op. cit., p. 88.

11. Sears, J.B. The Nature of Administrative Practice. New York, McGraw-Hill Book Company, 1950, pp. 7-14.

12. Ibid., pp. 550-551.

13. Leifer, op. cit., p. 25.

14. Stokes, G.A. The Roles Psychiatric Nurses in Community Mental Health Practice: A Giant Step. New York, Maimonides Medical Center—Community Mental Health Center, 1969, p. i.

DISCUSSION

Mr. Morse:

The difficulty in the decision-making process represents complex problems that have implications for nursing. As community mental health center practice moves from the medical model to an ecological model—the power must shift from a medical authority to a multidisciplinary group.

This reflects what is occurring in society at large. As we become a more technologically-oriented society, erosion in the primary family unit occurs; but, prior to this, the extended family has been disbanded, so that many of us have not experienced health primary group relationships. The urban area tends to attract people who have had an impoverished primary group relationship. Professional staff as well as the consumers of service have had a similar experience. We're people who may come from broken families, or from a small family, where we have not really learned to relate to a group or to simultaneous multiple relationships. If we are lucky, experientially, we get involved at some time in a group where we have to develop multiple relationships, rather than just relative to a single person. We have people coming into groups in the community mental health center who are not able to do this. Encounter groups and marathon groups were developed to help overcome these barriers. It is therefore not only a problem of the administrative structure, it's a problem of society.

Mr. Morse:

To me the essence of nursing is utilizing a relationship. All nurses may not agree with that, or even understand it or have the capability of using it. If people were to agree that the essence of nursing is the relationship, then the education would be different, and we would screen individuals who could benefit by the educational experience.

Comment:

As I see it, the issue is no longer whether or not to shift from the medical model to the ecological model; the issue is what the essence of the ecological model is. To me the ecological model includes a shift in focus from a mental illness to a *mental health model*, in other words, a shift from tertiary and secondary prevention to primary prevention. The mental health model is one which is concerned with the health needs of people in all life experiences rather than with crisis intervention only.

Mr. Morse:

It is *not* a shift in focus but a new way of conceptualizing and experiencing people within a system. The ecological model is a gestalt idea. It focuses on how we approach, assess, and intervene with individuals, groups, and the total community, working with the forces within and without.

Comment:

When we talk about change and social systems, an important thing is to look at what we want to change—or what is it that the public wants changed. We need to work with community groups in looking at the setting in which change is to occur. Some of these general terms do need to be clarified.

Mr. Morse:

When we talk about the issue of the medical model, there is an underlying theme or issue of authority. The medical model represents authority. In talking about giving it up, we have to deal with the issue of dependency and security versus independence and its consequence. An analogy may be drawn to the period of adolesence, and the relationship between parent and teenager. In talking about the center of power and the shifts that need to occur, theoretically the change has been made, but operationally change has not occurred. We are still struggling with a medically-dominated program.

Comment:

Perhaps we are not ready to relinquish the medical model wherein the doctor assumes responsibility. We are ambivalent about assuming responsibility for our own behavior; if we are able to assume responsibility and determine to do it—let's get on with it; if we need someone to tell us "you've got to do it," maybe we are not comfortable enough with our independence, ability or worth to give up the medical model. Then we must continue with it. There's a certain security in knowing what the medical model is—and that it's there. We can always say that it's awful and we hate it, and things like that. If it were not there, then we would be really very much accountable for our own practice and behavior, and the community would force nurses to be accountable, not only to themselves, but to the community; this could sometimes be very uncomfortable.

On the other hand it doesn't really matter what kind of model you are working with. If you are a professional—which implies that you are accountable—it does not matter what your organizational structure is, you're still accountable for what *you* do. Therefore, the model is not the issue; the issue is accountability or, change and risk. Yes, I am accountable for myself, to my patients, to the community mental health board, and to my agency, pretty much in that order, by my own decision. I worked out that order of accountability for myself.

Question:

In talking about responsiveness to the community, I'm wondering if we're not viewing "community" in different ways. Are you equating community mental health boards—that is, a politically appointed official agency—with the community—that is, its people?

Comment:

Yes, our community mental health board is a county board, an official board elected by the people of the community and is not run by any officer of any institution or by any governor. The community residents have the power to say whether or not you can practice in their community—whether or not you get a salary. They actually review everyone who is to work in their community and determine whether he may work there. Furthermore, if you do not continue to earn the right they can relieve you of your responsibilities and salary.

Question:

Who sets up the machinery so that they have this power?

Comment:

The machinery evolved from a coalition group of all the health services in the community. This group existed before our agency was created. The community mental health board determines the priorities of services that we give–for example, we were asked to provide services for children, adolescents, and the elderly specifically in the areas of addiction and community organization. Remember this–the impetus for establishing the community mental health center came from the people in the community. They were the ones who petitioned for funds and then turned the actual work of writing the grant over to the professionals.

Comment:

Various community people have different kinds of involvement. The impetus for establishing our community mental health center came from the professionals–the medical and social work administrators, and the nursing director who went out into the community and tried to get people in the community involved. When the adjoining community heard about our mental health center, the people in the community, many of whom were professional, assembled and discussed the lack of comparable services and went into action. Subsequently, those community people as a group sought the support of their state senator who went to the funding agency–to the county community mental health board, and developed a community mental health center in the area. The impetus came from them, and they are really involved. A budget was developed and a psychiatrist appointed. They were the ones who, along with the advisory staff from our center, interviewed and appointed the psychiatrist, and now every single person who is going to be hired will be interviewed by the psychiatrist, who will be the director, and by the community people. The community people are now looking for a location for the center.

Comment:

Community involvement occurs in different ways and on different levels. It seems to me that there might be more community involvement if the initial step comes from the grassroots.

Question:

Does this really make a difference in terms of our responsibility to the community? Shouldn't we be meeting the needs of the community, whether a community mental health service was founded by the people or imposed on them?

Comment:

That's a tricky one–you're talking in an idealistic sense. My first thought is, where is the pressure coming from? In a larger system, it may be that you respond to the person who actually doesn't have the greatest pressure – for instance your immediate supervisor–or your director. In a large system you get insulated from the community because you are surrounded by that system.

Comment:

I don't think that's necessarily true. I work in an agency which is very large—almost too large to be called a community mental health center. Three agencies work under one roof, and they function separately, so that there are a lot of direct supervisors and indirect supervisors, and a large organizational structure—but the pressure is coming directly from the community, and we can feel it. The service was started originally by a small group of people who went out and demonstrated the need, accumulated money from private trust funds, and then approached the city to share the expenses of starting a hospital for the medically indigent in the city. We then had two groups representing the private and the public sector. Then the state initiated the mental health center. From the time the private group convened and originated the idea, and accumulated the money, the philosophy of a community-oriented hospital treating psychiatric disorders of the medically indigent, remained constant, even though it was an inpatient service prior to the development of the community mental health center. Originally there was not too much pressure from the recipients of the service, because service had never been provided before. However, now we are getting pressure from them, as they demand "more." People assembled in the lobby and informed us of their needs. We have a steering committee made up of black people from organizations that represent the black community. Each organization is represented by an elected member from passive organizations as well as from the Black Panthers. The committee sets priorities and we respond in order or priority, within the limits of the budget. They are aware of budget limitations on the services and they are willing to help. For instance, with the development of a drug abuse program we couldn't provide the amount of service needed as we didn't have the staff or the space; so they secured space and helped us with staff by volunteering their people. Together, we developed how much we could do, and they, in turn, helped to expand the services required.

Comment:

The needs of the community should determine the priority and the kinds of services. If, however, federal funding provides a comprehensive community mental health center, the five federally required services must be offered, otherwise you lose the federal allocation. The community must be informed regarding these external forces. The service within the governmental mandates is a shared community endeavor.

Question:

We have been discussing the organized elements in the community, what about the needs of the unorganized clients?

Comment:

You pursue them. You bring them to the center, and you listen to them. One of our groups expressed dissatisfaction saying, "Some of the treatment we get is very impersonal and when we go to the center, all the people want to do is give us medication and so we stop going to the center." We tried to personalize the services so that our clients realize that giving medication isn't all we want to do.

In responding to the community however, we don't always respond to their satisfaction. For example, in responding to the police force, we may antagonize them, and our responses to the courts at times are not exactly what they want, and these are two important parts of the community. I take the position that unless we take a stand on issues, we cannot function in the community setting.

Question:

From your response, I conclude that you are not advocating community control?

Comment:

Not totally. I think that would be an abdication of the professional's responsibility. You can only respond to the part of the community with whom you have dialogue. If we are the experts, we have an obligation to outline alternatives. There are many people in need of care that do not verbalize the need and these people are not represented. They may be alcoholics, they may be retired people, they may be people with problems they believe are unique, and about which they cannot talk. We need to be responsive to the people who express their needs but we also need to identify the unexpressed needs that exist in the community, otherwise, the most vociferous and energetic people are going to get the attention, and the silent ones will remain neglected.

Comment:

The theme of the discussions so far is: how do we share power? When we talk about the traditional medical model, the power is in the medical model and not in the community. On the other hand, in the programs where clients are involved in decision-making, power *is* in the community; the problem between black and white is a question of sharing of power; the relationship of nurses with other disciplines is a problem of sharing power. Decision-making is sharing power. Functioning in a complex administrative structure represents an attempt to share power.

The Nurse's Role in Planning Inner-City Mental Health Services

ANITA L. NARCISO, R.N., M.S.

The legendary Phoenix, a beautiful female bird, was fabled to live for five hundred years, to build herself a funeral pyre and fanning the flames with her wings to be consumed by her own act and to arise in youthful freshness from these ashes to begin her life cycle again.

Entrepreneurs of "Model Cities Programs" and some of the torch-bearing activists from the inner city have similar dreams of Baltimore rising from the ashes of her own social revolution to begin a new life cycle. In Baltimore, the fire is fanned by a very high crime rate, a high incidence of drug abuse, and the highest homicide rate in the nation. Simultaneously, the flames are fanned by conflicting cultures, high mobility, great poverty, family disorganization, and much personal insecurity.

It is a recognized concept that the rate of mental disorganization is highest when a group of people are put in the position of desiring certain ends—ends that society in general regards as possible and desirable for everyone—and yet are prevented by the organization of society from being able to realize those ends.[1]

Faris and Dunham found that, in Chicago, increased rates of schizophrenia occurred among hoboes, rooming house occupants, persons foreign born, and Negroes, living in the central business district. The lowest rates occurred among native-born living in the residential and high-rental apartment house districts.[2]

The same pattern holds true in Baltimore. In comparison with the rest of the state of Maryland, Baltimore has the highest rate of admissions to state mental hospitals, totalling approximately 60 percent of admissions to all hospitals.[3] A study of admissions to the state mental hospitals, conducted over a six-month period in 1968, revealed that the greatest number of patients admitted resided in the downtown or transitional zone of Baltimore.

Metropolitan Baltimore comprises one area serviced by one of the six Regional Mental Health offices for the state Department of Mental Hygiene. This office is staffed by one psychiatrist who is also the Associate Director of Mental Health, Baltimore City Health Department. Recognizing the magnitude of his responsibility, the Associate Director initiated a request for additional professional staff, and received a state grant to the Baltimore City Health Department, Bureau of Public Health Nursing, to create the position of Community Mental Health Liaison Nurse.

Organizationally, the position was to be that of a staff specialist in the vertical structure of the Bureau of Public Health Nursing. Functionally, the position was to be that of liaison agent, specifically in the area of psychiatric nursing, between the Regional Mental Health Director for Baltimore City and the Bureau of Public Health Nursing. To enhance the liaison, the nurse would operate from the office of the Regional Mental Health Director for Baltimore City.

As a recipient of the state grant, I found myself in the unusual position of defining my own role within the limitations of five global objectives defined in the state grant: liaison, referral, consultation, teaching, and therapy. The role developed initially into one of reconciling the multiple demands of a group of social and health agencies that had been offered a new service. It soon became evident that the strongest basis for social power for the liaison nurse was in the effective quality of that role.

LIAISON FUNCTIONS

Specifically, as the catalyst-role of the liaison nurse became more evident among agency staffs (some of whom had never met or discussed mutual problems, programs, or goals), it was necessary to organize the multiphasic services of these agencies within the major catchment areas serviced by three of the state mental hospitals. Roughly, each of these hospitals is responsible for one-third of the total city population. By dividing the city in this manner, a basis for the coordination of the activities of these agencies was made clear.

At the same time, a closer relationship was developed among the nursing personnel of all three state mental hospitals and the district public health nurses located in the hospitals catchment areas. To further this closer relationship, a program has been developed by the directors of nursing of the state mental hospitals and the community mental health liaison nurse whereby selected nursing personnel of the state hospitals are introduced to the personnel and programs of the health and welfare agencies servicing the catchment area covered by the particular employing institution. The purpose of this program is to familiarize individuals with the process and mechanics of the involved intradisciplinary agencies.

As an outgrowth of the above program, an interagency referral form was developed as a formal means of communication. The creation of this form represents this adaptiveness which is inherent in highly complex organizations.[4] Creating the referral form was mutually beneficial both to the agents and agencies involved and, further, it represents the pragmatic nature of the role of the community mental health liaison nurse.

Most of the above organizations are bureaucratic in nature—that is, they constitute forms of closed systems in our political form of government. In themselves, the staff functions of a community mental health liaison nurse are a form of open system that permits the liaison nurse to receive information (data, if you will) and then process this information into useable data for the next level in the organization. In my role, I have been invited into every level of the state and city health departments, thus increasing the possibility of bridging many communication gaps.

The interagency referral form previously mentioned depicts the concept of tertiary prevention as described by Caplan.[5] It has become a functional tool when individual patients about to be discharged from state mental hospitals are referred to the public health nurse for support and greater utilization of outpatient clinic services.

The description of the program is a simplification—in fact, an oversimplification—of the role of entrepreneur that has gradually incorporated itself into the five stated areas of interest for the community mental health liaison nurse. As described by Filley and House, some of the characteristics of the entrepeneur are now inherent in my position.[6] The relative value of each new program has so outweighed the negative aspects that the fear of failure has been minimized by the need for achievement.

The charisma that goes with success has been transferred to some conservative members of involved organizations resulting in greater output. And, as Hage points out, "When the outputs are services to clients rather than manufacturing products, the organization is apt to show more adaptiveness, because there is less opportunity for standardization of tasks."[7] This has been particularly true with some of the conservative staff members of the Bureau of Public Health Nursing who have adapted to the team concept for providing continuous and contiguous nursing services to larger catchment areas. The concept of a concerted group effort had been alien to those individualists who had carried large catchment areas alone.

THE PROCESS OF CHANGE

Here again, involvement in the *process* of change has been the dynamic force for individual behavioral change. Once more the "flair for the game" of the

SPRINGFIELD STATE HOSPITAL INTER-AGENCY REFERRAL FORM

SEPARATION DATE   Address Where Patient Will Live   Home Phone _____

_____   _____   Emergency Phone _____

Clinic Appointment Date   _____   Soc. Sec. # _____

_____   Diagnosis: _____

__ Appointment Card
__ Given to Patient   Established __ Impression __   Education _____

MEDICATION ON RELEASE: No. of Hospital Admissions ___

                                   Occupation _____   FINANCIAL STATUS:
                                                                      __ D.S.S.   __ Pension
                                   ESTIMATED EMPLOYMENT STATUS: __ Medicare __ Other (Specify)
                                   __ Full Time
                                   __ Part Time   _____
                                   __ Able to Work
                                   __ Student, Housewife, etc.   KNOWN TO SOCIAL SERVICE
__ Medication Given   __ Retired   __ Yes   __ No
_____   __ Supportive Conditions Only   _____
CONDITION ON RELEASE: NOT EMPLOYABLE   FOLLOW-UP TREATMENT PLAN:
__ Recovered   __ Too Ill Physically   __ Outpatient Psychiatric
__ Improved   __ Too Ill Mentally   Clinic (Specify)
__ Unimproved   __ Too Ill Physical & Mental
__ No Mental Disorder   __ Other (Specify)   __ Private Psychiatrist
__ Legally Competent   __ Private Physician
__ Legally Incompetent   _____   __ Hospital Facility
__ Minor   PROGNOSIS: __ Psychiatric Day Care Center
                                   __ Poor   __ Nursing Home
_____   __ Good   __ Public Health Nurse
SEPARATION STATUS: __ Guarded   __ Clergy
__ Trial Visit   _____   __ Alcoholics Anonymous
__ Convalescent Leave   SOCIAL ENVIRONMENT: __ Special School
__ Foster Care   __ Lives Alone   __ Vocational Rehabilitation
__ Elopement   __ With Spouse   __ Legal Involvement (Specify)
__ Discharge   __ Foster Home
__ Transfer   __ With Relatives   __ Other (Specify)
__ Against Medical Advice   __ Other (Specify)   __ None

_____
                              MEDICAL DATA:
              Results and Date of Last: General Physical Condition and Comments:
Urinalysis _ _ _ _ _ _ _ _ _ _ _ _ _ _   __ Epileptic   __ Diabetic   __ Cardiac
C.B.C. _ _ _ _ _ _ _ _ _ _ _ _ _ _ _ _   __ Other (Specify) _ _ _ _ _ _ _ _ _ _ _ _
Blood Chemistry _ _ _ _ _ _ _ _ _ _ _ _   _
Chest X-ray _ _ _ _ _ _ _ _ _ _ _ _ _ _   _
_____
COMMENTS: (Include any pertinent information, evaluation, recommendation not covered
          above)

_____
Charge Ward Nurse Signature

_____
Hospital Ward Physician Signature   ADDRESSOGRAPH PLATE
SSH C-1

entrepreneur was instrumental in affecting my various roles as consultant, teacher, and therapist as each became situationally appropriate.

Because of the close working relationship between city agencies, the school department, city hospitals, public health agencies, and community action agencies, frequent requests for help and direction are referred to me. Over a period of time, the nature of these calls has changed. Initially, requests were specific in relation to individual clients of these various agencies and, frequently, the liaison aspect of my role in linking up interdependent functions of one or more agencies was all that was necessary. My superiors also pointed out to me that many of the requests in fact were testing mechanisms that had to be initiated before trusting relationships could be developed.

That phase of my "apprenticeship" seems to be completed as the nature of these requests usually are now directed toward assisting various members of agency staffs to become more sensitive to the needs of their clients. Only occasionally are the calls for assistance those which involve crisis intervention or individual personal problems, and the emerging role of the liaison nurse is now approaching my concept of the role of the nursing consultant in mental hygiène.

An example of this emerging role is seen in the conduct of group sessions with the counselors of the Neighborhood Youth Corps Program-Community Action Agency. My role here has been one of direct consultation, offering specific solutions, more acceptable in this socioeconomic framework, to problems presented by counselors. As the counselor sees them, the strengths of the individual clients are developed. The counselor is helped to focus on the client's presenting problems and to see himself as a positive agency of change.

Another example of my emerging role has grown out of the request to review and revise the curriculum used in an alcoholism training program for nurses and other professional groups through the Inner City Community Mental Health Center. This program is sponsored by the University of Maryland and has been beneficial for public health nurses to the extent that they have requested the assistance of an alcoholism counselor to provide casework coverage. My secondary role in this project has been to coordinate the services of an alcoholism counselor, who operates from the Southern Police District, with the services of the Southern District Public Health Nurse—services that have proved mutually beneficial to all concerned.

The administrative processes of planning, organizing, coordinating, controlling and evaluating, inherent in all programs, have been an integral part of my role. Primarily, my described functions have centered around the process of coordinating and evaluating existing programs, and planning activities usually have been centered around short-term goals.

Long-range planning and the implementation of an interdisciplinary project have brought about a change of focus in regard to the administrative process. At the request of the Police Department of the City of Baltimore, I was asked to assist in evaluating the system of transporting legally-committed patients to any of three state mental hospitals that service the city. As a result of a ruling by the State's Attorney, the responsibility for the transportation of mental and alcoholic patients has been delegated to the Department of Mental Hygiene.

The establishment of semi-autonomous units within a formal organizational structure like the Department of Mental Hygiene presents an opportunity for the individuals involved to independently create a small organization within the bureaucratic superstructure, and this occurred, essentially, when the transportation project was assigned to the office of the Regional Mental Health Director for Baltimore City. I then had the opportunity to promote a conceptual design I had helped innovate.

Since there was no precedent to follow, the design of the transportation unit was an outgrowth of the planning process and involved the areas of staffing, budgeting, logistical support, and supervision. Policies and the delegation of responsibility and authority were written within the framework of existing guidelines for the Department of Mental Hygiene. An evaluation tool, now being constructed, will complete the planning process.

LONG-RANGE PLANNING

The long-range planning aspects of this project, which is still in the design stage, project a receiving unit of 10 beds in a city hospital or a community mental health center. Expertise in a speciality area (in this case, knowledge about psychiatric nursing principles), has been my most effective tool in creating change in the long-range planning process. By incorporating the concept that case finding is a primary function of community mental health center, it has been possible, with the function of the transportation unit and the proposed receiving unit, to speak of an emerging pattern of psychiatric services for the City of Baltimore. This emerging pattern will provide coverage much like an umbrella held over the city, and will include six community mental health centers, the first of which already is operational in the inner city.

As Baltimore is emerging from its transitional stage, I find this a most challenging and useful time for involvement.

REFERENCES

1. Davis, K. Human Society. New York, the Macmillan Company, 1949, p. 277.
2. Faris, R., and Dunham, H. Mental Disorders in Urban Areas, an ecological study of schiozophrenia and other psychoses. Chicago, University of Chicago Press, 1939, pp. 38-57.
3. State Department of Mental Hygiene, Office of Planning, Progress Report and State Plan, 1969-1970, For Mental Health Services. Baltimore,

Maryland, June 1968, p. 8.

4. Hage, J. An axiomatic theory of organizations. Admin. Sci. Quart., 10:289-320, December, 1965.
5. Caplan, G. Principles of Preventive Psychiatry, New York, Basic Books, Inc., 1964, p. 26.
6. Filley, A., and House, R. Managerial Process and Organizational Behavior. Glenview, Illinois, Scott, Foresman and Company, 1969, p. 458.
7. Hage, J. op. cit. p. 305.

DISCUSSION

Question:

Which of the factors that brought about the grant application made your role possible?

Miss Narciso:

The need came out of the riots—the city fathers wanted to "cool the city." No real enthusiasm was evident about making real changes in the ghetto. However, changes have taken place in the ghetto since the April riots. These changes were brought about by our working collaboratively with community action groups through projects funded by the Office of Economic Opportunity. I had problems getting into some groups; I was accepted at first because our physician is black. Together, we helped to bring about some of the changes. We encouraged citizen participation—which became mandatory because we developed them as guidelines for the project proposal for funding. The citizens of the inner-city have formed a committee to make their needs known. We advocate the involvement of community people in advisory groups and in action groups in those areas where the need for change is most apparent. For example, the local hospital, which is located in a black community, wanted to provide community mental health services for the area. In addition, it was providing services to a new city located 25 miles away. The hospital was concentrating its services more on the new area than on the area surrounding the hospital. The black people in the community became aroused, called our office and we arranged a meeting. As a result of that meeting, the local hospital developed a drug abuse program for the teenagers because parents identified this as the prime need.

Question:

You mentioned wanting to renew the grant. Is this because you feel you could not function any other way in the bureaucratic structure?

Miss Narciso:

I have something going, and it's easier to bring about change by staying "open"—functioning between the two systems rather than getting boxed in.

Besides my preferences, it has to do with change theory. There is need to have several persons unite and pull together different kinds of agencies.

Question:

Your relationship with the nurses in the state hospital is of interest. How did you help the nurses to become motivated to move outside the state hospital walls?

Miss Narciso:

The nurses in the state hospital complained that 50 percent of their patients came from the inner city. So I went out to see what we could do. That was my entry to their setting. The hospital services are regionalized so that all the patients from the inner city are housed in one to three buildings. I met with the nurses as a group and asked them what they wanted us to do.

Most of the nurses lived at least 25 to 50 miles away in the suburban or rural areas and seldom visited the city. They were not familiar with what patients really had to deal with. They realized that they were getting many readmissions because of the lack of follow-up facilities. The hospital's outpatient departments were 25 miles away from the city, which created hardships; for example, it requires three buses and eight hours to get to an outpatient department for a 15-minute examination and a renewal of medication. The first thing that had to be done was to make the outpatient departments more accessible and refer some discharged patients to the public health nurses. Some of the nurses in the state hospital developed teams to function in the outpatient department, continued to see the same patients, and in addition, began to make home visits. These nurses have been instrumental in developing aftercare programs for patients.

Arrangements were made for the nurses to visit the housing projects where many of the patients were living. Their first reactions were: "The housing projects are beautiful—this wouldn't be a bad place to live." However, this was short-lived, as they soon encountered the odors, the delinquents, and other adversities that the resident had to tolerate. It was a very eye-opening experience for the nurses as they really became involved. The majority of them have remained involved with the community either in conducting groups or visiting patients and families in their houses to be certain that they don't lose touch with patients once they leave the hospital. A small number have restricted themselves to the hospital.

Question:

What kind of back-up or support do you provide for the public health nurses?

Miss Narciso:

I run an inservice education session twice a week for an hour-and-a-half. We have a three-point program: (1) didactic content—including psychiatric nursing and psychiatric theory. Many of the public health nurses had their basic nursing education before psychiatric nursing was an integral part of the program. The didactic material includes basic principles, plus case finding and case supervision. Each nurse selects a patient or family and we explore her ability to deal with the situation; (2) I sometimes do visiting with a nurse to provide support; and (3) nurses participate in a group-process training program so that they can move from the individual approach into a group setting where they work as a team. This program has been going on for about 18 months.

Question:

Are these public health nursing supervisors?

Miss Narciso:

No, they are staff nurses. Supervisors appear to be threatened by us, so the psychiatrist works with the supervisors. He has helped one supervisor leave who couldn't adapt to the changes. There have been innovative changes in oriented consultation. Their preference apparently stems from a fear that the doctor would interfere if he knew of their request for psychiatric nursing consultation. Generally, nursing administration is supportive and encouraging but unable to deal with the problems of interferences by the physician. There appears to be a lack of meaningful communication between the nursing and medical personnel at all levels.

Question:

What do you see as priority for a nurse in organizing and planning community mental health care?

Miss Narciso:

When a community is organizing for community mental health, the nurse needs to be in on the planning phase. She should get together with whoever else happens to be in there in order to get the necessary job done. There will be greater likelihood of good nursing input from the beginning. During planning you speak for nursing, the development of policy, and the provision of nursing input and nursing contributions.

Nurses definitely have a significant contribution to make in affecting change in the delivery of mental health services. What that contribution is depends on who the nurse is, where she is, how she sees herself, and within what geographical and organizational structure she functions. For example, we're trying to get the six community mental health centers to coordinate staff and money with state hospital personnel, so that state personnel could move in and out of the six community mental health centers, and the community mental health center personnel similarly could move in and out of the state hospital.

Ideally, there would be six joint teams. The problem is not only in crossing administrative policies and budgets, but in asking the superintendents of mental health care to give up some of their control. Community people are sometimes viewed negatively.

An important corollary of this is that the nurse who participates in planning either helps the group to listen directly to the community, or at least becomes an advocate for the community because many nurses are where they can see what the needs are face-to-face. For example, a drug abuse program for teenagers, or care for disturbed children, or help with an alcoholic spouse.

Question:

I am concerned with the steps taken before a program is planned. How can you plan for a community until you really know what that community is all about?

Comment:

I agree with you. I don't see how you can help a community plan community services without having the community in on the planning. This is the crux of the situation. A nurse must understand the problems and be able to project herself so that she is invited to the citizens' meetings.

Comment:

Nurses must speak for nursing and not have someone else speak for it. You know that we're saying the same thing when we state that nurses are advocates for the community. . . . The community should be involved in speaking for itself in the initial planning stages.

The Role of the Nurse in the Development of Local Services Within a Statewide Mental Health Plan

SARAH HELEN CARLTON, R.N., M.N.

The Community Mental Health Centers Act of 1963 provided the impetus for the development of community mental health centers throughout the country by providing funds for the construction and staffing of these centers. In Florida, in the last three years, eight comprehensive community mental health centers have been established to provide the indicated essential services, and five more centers are in varying stages of development. Communities and centers in our state have faced many problems in the process of developing a comprehensive program. Many of the difficulties center around the philosophical understanding and commitment of the mental health professionals toward developing a comprehensive program. Another problem is the shortage of professional manpower to implement services.[1] Both the shortage of professionals and the expansion of the traditional treatment resources in a community has led to enlargement of the traditional roles of the mental health professionals. A departure from traditional roles has created different reactions among the professionals, depending on the degree of comfort the particular professional feels with change, his own philosophy about how mental health needs can be met most effectively, and his ideas about how he fits into meeting those needs. Thus, the role of a professional in a community mental health program is determined by the individual, as well as by the needs of the community the program serves.

As is true in other disciplines, the role of a nurse in a comprehensive community mental health center is dependent on many factors, including those of both an external and internal nature. External factors include the community needs, the receptivity of the community to attempted fulfillment of these needs, and the administrative environment of the center which determines the degree of freedom the nurse has to develop her role and also determines the effective atmosphere of relationships among disciplines. Some of the most important internal factors include the nurse's educational and professional background, her individual concept of what community mental health nursing is, her ability to identify her role in a certain center program, and her own reactions to external role determinants.

According to Virginia Henderson, "The unique function of the nurse is to assist the individual, sick or well, in the performance of those activities contributing to health or its recovery (or to peaceful death) that he would perform unaided if he had the necessary strength, will or knowledge. And to do this in such a way as to help him gain independence as rapidly as possible. It is my contention that the nurse is, and should be legally, an independent practitioner and able to make independent judgments as long as he, or she, is not diagnosing, prescribing treatment for disease, or making a prognosis, for these are the physician's functions."[2-3] Community mental health nursing demands that the nurse be able to function independently in a variety of settings, as well as able to collaborate with other disciplines, other agencies, and other nurses.

The nurse in a community mental health center program is often faced with a specific problem. More often than not, people in other mental health disciplines are not knowledgeable about how the nurse is able to function outside a medical, hospital-oriented program and it is largely up to the nurse to demonstrate her functions. Her ability to do this is related to her own comfort, both personally and professionally, in a situation where she has minimal direction and often is received with doubt and resistance. On the other hand, community mental health nursing has many opportunities for a nurse to expand her interests and skills, to grow professionally as a result of her contact with a variety of people in other disciplines and agencies, and to utilize her specific talents. In short, the nurse has the opportunity to "do her thing" in community mental health.

CLINICAL EXPERIENCES

I will attempt now to make some generalizations about the role of a nurse-clinical specialist in a community mental health center program, based on some of my experiences in a newly-developing program in Panama City, Florida. The comprehensive program in this community is provided by two separate facilities, located across the street from each other. One, the general hospital, received funds for the construction of inpatient, emergency, and day treatment facilities, the construction was completed and put into actual operation in January, 1968. The Guidance Clinic, which had already been established in the community, expanded its services to include (in addition to outpatient services), education and consultation, precare and aftercare, diagnostic, rehabilitative, and training services. Prior to the construction of inpatient facilities in the community, inpatient care was sought in the state hospital, about 80 miles away, or by private treatment in a city about 100 miles away.

The catchment area served by the center covers a predominantly rural, six-county area in northwest Florida, with a population of approximately 150,000. The center is located in the center of population and is within 60 miles of the northern-most county seats. There are two satellite guidance clinics being established, one in the secondary population center in a northern county and another in a southern county. The area is characterized by families of low socioeconomic status, social and cultural deprivation, and an ultra-conservative attitude toward education, change and, specifically, treatment for mental health problems. The people in the northern half of the area make their living by farming; in the southern half of the area the largest industries are forestry and fishing.

The tourist trade is the largest "business" in the Panama City area because of the beaches. Also located in the Panama City area is an Air Force base, Naval base, and Naval research laboratory. Thus, the population in Panama City is a relatively transient and varied population. Mental illness, as can be predicted with such a population, is a number one health problem, ranking first in the rate of admissions per 100,000 population to state mental hospitals throughout the state.[4]

I joined the center program several months before the inpatient unit and day treatment center had been completed in the hospital portion. At that time there were two nurse-clinical specialist positions available, one in the hospital and one in the guidance clinic. The hospital had the greatest need for a nurse, and (at that time), my interest in the hospital position was greater. In the hospital setting I saw the opportunity to help start a new program, select and train staff, and carry the primary responsibility for developing the therapeutic program in collaboration with the two psychiatrists.

I also saw the opportunity to help educate the general hospital personnel about mental health and the goals of our program, to get involved in direct patient care, to work with families and groups, and to involve community agencies and interest groups in the program. These were some of the opportunities I could not afford to ignore. Also, I was able to foresee some of the problems that I would face. Most important of these was the tremendous task ahead in developing a truly therapeutic program which would provide an atmosphere for the patient to improve, an education for the general hospital staff about the mental health program, and the challenge of dealing with an enormous amount of resistance to the program.

Fortunately, I was provided in the beginning with a great deal of individual freedom and support from the hospital administration. Four months before the inpatient unit actually opened, I began selecting the staff and initiated the inservice education program. This period provided an opportunity for both the skeletal staff and me to learn to work together as a group; it provided a situation where I could share my personal ideas about mental health and caring for the mentally ill person with the staff, and it provided the staff the opportunity to work through many of their fears and feelings about mental patients. I covered the basic psychotherapeutic nursing skills and, when possible, the students used the existing clinical situation with the general hospital patients serving as a laboratory for practice. For example, as I covered the basic skills in interviewing, the students were given interview assignments with medical or surgical patients, which gave them an opportunity to relate to the general hospital staff and increase communication.

After the inpatient unit opened, one of my major responsibilities continued to be staff development, both formal and informal. Weekly inservice programs were offered during which staff were encouraged to assume responsibility for the content by means of clinical presentations and their theoretical application. Informal staff development took place in the form of daily team meetings for each shift during which individual patient care was planned and specific patient or staff problems were dealt with. Each team member—nurse, psychiatric aide or technician, housekeeper, ward clerk, or dietetic consultant—was encouraged to identify his particular contribution to patient care. These team meetings provided me with the opportunity to delegate much of the responsibility for patient care and to supervise the team in a group—which seemed most practical, considering the amount of other administrative responsibility I carried. Education and group supervision were important aspects of my role with the staff, which would seem to apply to the role of nurses in similar positions in other mental health programs.

The experiences I had with the staff (between 30 and 40 people employed at any one time), are some of the most rewarding experiences I had in the hospital. Initially, and throughout the 18 months in that position, my role with the staff was very similar to that of a teacher and role-model, encouraging each staff member to assume responsibility and to seek assistance when necessary. My relationship with the staff was a most unusual one and seemed to be one in which learning did occur. This was quite different from the normal supervisory relationships in the general hospital, however, and often produced problems with other nurses and the administration. Loomis states that the clinical specialist can "improve and influence nursing care given by the staff nurses and thus participate in the treatment of more patients than would be possible if she were functioning independently."[5] Generally, this seems to be applicable to nursing in any of the service elements in a community mental health center where a nurse is working with and through groups.

Other responsibilities that influenced my role in the hospital can be broken down into those of a strictly clinical and those of an administrative nature. Clinical responsibilities included getting involved in direct patient care, working with families, carrying a large responsibility for working with groups as well as assisting other staff members to do this, and participation in community meetings. Administrative responsibilities included planning and implementing the overall therapeutic program through collaboration with the psychiatrists, and utilizing a consultative relationship with the guidance clinic. In general, our program was set up as a therapeutic community and many of the activities involved getting the patient out into the community and bringing the community into the hospital.

The administrative responsibilities proved to be the most frustrating of all my hospital experiences. Often I was in a position of being responsible for the program but unable to carry out the responsibility because of lack of the necessary authority to accomplish this. In my position, I often served as the liaison person between the physicians and hospital administration—another difficult task. In essence, the therapeutic community environment in the mental health unit was most difficult to accomplish because of an already existing authoritarian power structure. However, in general, the program was sound and was able to withstand, for the most part, the periods of confusion.

THE GUIDANCE CLINIC

After my 18 months with the hospital program, I decided to accept the position with the guidance clinic and became involved in the other facets of the center's program. The guidance clinic has a staff of 14 professionals comprising a combination of disciplines including four psychologists, a reading therapist, a pastoral counselor, two consulting psychiatrists, three social workers—one of whom does precommitment investigations through the county judge's office—a mental health representative, and myself, a nurse.

The pervading philosophy in the clinic, allowing for much individual freedom for each person to develop his role, encourages a person to utilize his special skill in a variety of mental health services. There seems to be little concern about traditional roles, and emphasis is placed on staff members becoming generalists as well as specialists in their own area of mental health work. Blurring of roles and overlapping of functions is common. The flexible atmosphere has served to increase common elements of concern in the professionals and to encourage communication; hence, interdisciplinary relationships are comfortable. This is not to say, however, that duplication of service occurs. In my varied experiences at the clinic, my nursing orientation has broadened greatly and I have been made to feel that I make a special contribution to the program because of my specialty and my particular interests. The comfort that I have felt in this atmosphere has allowed me to grow personally and also has freed me professionally to develop my potential more fully.

In a recent study of the nurse's role in outpatient clinics in the United States, Holmes and Werner found that nurses functioned in varying capacities ranging from clinic receptionists to therapists.[6] In the last decade there has been much debate about whether or not a nurse would "do" therapy and to what extent she should assume the role of "therapist." Part of the reluctance of nurses to do therapy seems to be bound up with that stone wall of tradition, and with the physician-nurse relationship in a medically-oriented program; it is also a question of semantics. According to Peplau, nurses can't hide much longer behind the general notion that they shouldn't do therapy, "for if the professional nurse doe not become an active participant in psychotherapeutic work, someone else will."[7]

Regardless of what it is called, nurses do assist people in learning to cope with their problems of living and nurses can provide experiences for people which will enhance this ability to cope. Caplan feels that the nurse is sociologically and psychologically close to the patient—and his family—in both space and time and sees the nurse as a particularly effective person on the mental health team.[8] This is certainly true of the nurse in the hospital setting, because the nurse is the only professional that maintains a continuous relationship with the patient. The public health nurse, having already been identified as a community helper, has easy access to the home.[9] Caplan is concerned about prevention of illness as well as providing assistance to the whole family with a medical problem. The nurse therefore is in a very enviable position since she is able to assist the mental health patient and his family during hospitalization, to prevent the need for rehospitalization by her early recognition of problems and her psychotherapeutic intervention when recurrent problems arise, and to promote mental health itself.[10] In addition to providing treatment resources that are easily accessible to people in the community, one of the goals of the community mental health center is the prevention of mental illness.[11] It follows that the public health resource should be tapped and assisted by the mental health professionals to do what it is already doing.

In my position with the guidance clinic I have been given freedom to develop my role according to my interests and the community's needs. One of my major contributions has been in developing the aftercare program in the six-county catchment area for people who have been hospitalized (usually in the state hospital) and then returned to the community. In all of the counties except one, once a person is released, the public health nurse is responsible for the aftercare on referrals received from the state hospital. The extent of the followup care varies from county to county, but almost always does include providing medication to the indigent patient. In some of the more economically prosperous counties in our catchment area the followup consists of regular home visits and consultation with the physician about the patient's medication. There is a great need to provide more comprehensive followup for these patients and their families and to provide assistance to the public health nurses in dealing with the mental health caseload.

Since I have a personal interest in working with psychotics in remission and with hardcore families, and because of my interest in nursing, I accepted the responsibility to develop a more comprehensive aftercare program by setting up regular consultation with the public health nurses and by providing a new service, a group therapy situation available to patients in each of the communities. A public health nurse is involved as a co-therapist in these groups. The assistance I have provided has been tailored to each individual county, but generally has taken the form of working with groups of nurses and groups of patients. In both instances group work was done because of the economical factor involved as well as my own preference of working with groups rather than individuals.

The group consultation approach is a helping as well as an educational and growth-producing process. The consultant makes use of group process and the consultees' personal involvement in their work problems.[12] From my own experience, it would seem that the psychiatric nurse in a center program could make a contribution in terms of planning and coordinating the followup care with the care received by the patient while in the hospital.

OTHER RESPONSIBILITIES

In addition to my responsibilities in the aftercare program, I am involved in consulting on a monthly basis with special education teachers in four of the counties, and in working with individuals and families in crisis intervention; I also spend time in individual long- and short-term psychotherapy with adolescents and adults, and in marital counseling. Recently I established a group for patients in a nursing home in the community and a group for adults in the guidance clinic. There is a need for more group treatment situations in the clinic programs, and since I am particularly interested in group work, I am attempting to meet this need.

My role in the guidance clinic has been a matter of self determination, identifying needs in the program and utilizing my interests and skill to attempt to meet these needs. The same thing would apply for a nurse or any other professional in any elements of a community mental health center program.

In summary, I think it will be helpful to compare and contrast the role I have assumed in the two different settings in our community mental health center. First, I am impressed by their similarity, particularly in the area of the type of services with which I have become involved. In both programs (hospital and guidance clinic) I have focused my attention on developing or expanding services where a gap in services has existed. I have been most concerned with developing the program around the community and in utilizing community resources. I have worked as a change agent with professional and staff groups and thus have provided indirect services to patients. My major interest has been in group work with patients and, although both settings have provided many opportunities for working with groups, the focus of groups in the two settings has differed.

In the hospital setting, treatment was short-term in nature and often consisted of crisis intervention. People who needed followup care and long-term treatment were referred to the guidance clinic. The psychiatrist assumed the primary responsibility for the treatment, and the staff was utilized in a therapeutic role. The mental health program in the hospital has met with much resistance from hospital personnel, including physicians, nurses, the staffs of other departments in the hospital, and the administration. Much of this resistance was focused on such things as whether the staff should wear street clothes or uniforms. The basis of the resistance seemed to reflect a generalized negative attitude toward the community mental health program and the use of federal funds for the development of such a program. This hospital atmosphere seemed to reflect the typical reaction of an ultra-conservative community in this section of the state. Regardless of the cause of the resistance, the mental health program has had much difficulty in maintaining itself in this particular hospital setting.

The Guidance Clinic has faced fewer problems and part of this is due to the fact that the clinic has been in existence in the community for a number of years. It has been an expanded rather than a totally new and different program. The treatment philosophy of the clinic is focused on a multidisciplinary approach, with the various mental health professions such as psychology, psychiatry, social work, and nursing assuming independent and collaborative therapeutic roles.

As a psychiatric nurse, I have been involved in long-term therapy in addition to crisis intervention and short-term therapy with clients. The administrative atmosphere in the Guidance Clinic has been more comfortable, and I believe this atmosphere is the prime attribute in terms of role development. In other words, the *affective* atmosphere constitutes the major difference in the two experiences.

BIBLIOGRAPHY

Bulbuyan, A. Dividites, R.M., Williams, F. Nurses in community mental health centers. Amer. J. Nurs., 69:328-331, Feb., 1969.

Caplan, G. An Approach to Community Mental Health, New York, Grune & Stratton, Inc., 1961.

Eisendorfer, C., Altrocchi, J., and Young F. Principles of community mental health in a rural setting: the Halifax county program. Commun. Ment. Health Jour., 4:211-220, June, 1968.

Hankoff, L.D., Bernabo, L.B., and Omura, J. Visiting nurse consultation in a

community psychiatry program. J. Psych. Nurs., 5:217-232, May–June, 1967.
Hess, G. Perception of the nursing role in a developing mental health center. J. Psych. Nurs., 7:77-81, March-April, 1969.
Holmes, J., and Werner, J.A. Psychiatric Nursing in a Therapeutic Community. New York, The Macmillan Company, 1966.
Mereness, D. The potential significant role of the nurse in community mental health services. Persp. Psych. Care, 1:34-39, May-June-July, 1969.
Messick, J.M., and Aguilera, D.C. A schema: the psychiatric nurse on the community mental health team. J. Psych. Nurs., 5:431-439, September-
October, 1966. Sheldon, A., and Hope, P. K. The developing role of the nurse in a community mental health program. Persp. Psych. Care, 5:272-279, 1969.
Stretch, J.J. Community mental health: the evolution of a concept of social policy. Comm. Men. Health, 3:5-12, Spring 1967.
Walkon, G.H. Effecting a continuum of care: an exploitation of the crisis of hospital release. Commun. Ment. Health J., 4:63-73, February, 1968.
Wray, E.O. Crisis intervention-a nursing role in community mental health programs. J. Psych. Nurs. 3:394-400, September–October, 1965.

REFERENCES

1. Joint Commission on Mental Illness and Health. Action for Mental Health, New York, Science Editions, Inc., 1961, p. 140.
2. Henderson, V. The Nature of Nursing: A Definition of Its Implications for Practice, Research, and Education. New York, The MacMillan Company, 1966, p. 15.
3. Ibid., p. 16.
4. Division of Mental Health, Department of Community Mental Health. Florida State Plan for the Construction of Community Mental Health Centers, 1969, p. 45.
5. Loomis, E. The clinical specialist as a change agent. Nurs. Forum, 7:136, 1968.
6. Reres, M.E. A survey of the nurse's role in psychiatric outpatient clinics in America. Commun. Ment. Health J., 5:382-385, Oct., 1969.
7. Peplau, H. Psychotherapy and the Professional Nurse. Speech given at Neuropsychiatric Institute, University of California Medical Center, Los Angeles, California, July 2, 1964.
8. Caplan, G. Principles of Preventive Psychiatry. New York, Basic Books, Inc., 1964.
9. Ujhely, G.B. The nurse in community psychiatry. Amer. J. Nurs., 69:1001-1005, May, 1969.
10. Peplau, H. The nurse in the community mental health program. Nurs. Outlook, 68-70, Nov., 1965.
11. Joint Commission on Mental Illness and Health, op. cit., p. 208.
12. Altrocchi, J., Spielberger, C.C., and Eisendorfer, C. Mental health consultation with groups. Commun. Ment. Health J., I:127:134, Summer, 1965.

DISCUSSION

Question:
Could you tell us more about the problem of resistance, what and how you were able to work around this problem?

Miss Carlton:
There is an ultraconservative attitude among the community people toward mental illness, mental health professionals, mental health education and even toward change. Although I believe my attitude is different, I can understand their problems—having grown up in northwest Florida. Initially there was support from the hospital administrators. The task was to plan and implement therapeutic programs four months before the unit opened. I was getting to know nurses, physicians and was able to select staff. In the beginning, the director of nurses referred outstanding people—both professional and paraprofessional—to me. A skeletal staff spent one and a half hours a day for four months lashing out feelings about mental illness and how to help those in need. This planning period allowed the group to acquire basic psychiatric nursing knowledge and skills such as interviewing. It also provided opportunity to relate to the general hospital staff, increase communication with them, recruit, and spread the word. The psychiatrist was willing to meet with me one hour a week over lunch for consultation regarding the therapeutic program. He would say, "Now, you know more about community mental health programs, so you set it up—that'll be fine with us." This was nice in one way. I'd set it up, always trying to get their ideas. However, often they were reluctant to share and, in the end, we'd have to undo the whole thing.

As we progressed, there were other problems stemming from the hospital staff. They were concerned about the effect of building a new unit with federal funds. There was resistance from all disciplines, things like avoiding or coming late to group meetings. I think that they believe it represented giving away medical care when it ought to be bought. There was some fear of federal control over the center program.

In addition, my role in inservice education in the hospital was suspect to the hospital administration. Several years ago the nurses had received help from the American Nurses' Association and, as a result, their salaries had to be increased. Subsequently, inservice or any kind of group activity was not well thought of as it meant nurses could get together and talk about their problems and, collectively, do something about them. The hospital feared social action inside the hospital. However, I continued my efforts, working as a change-agent and influencing others. The hospital started its own inservice program and hired a director of inservice education. After the inpatient unit opened, it became one of my major responsibilities. As I said previously, the administrative responsibilities were the most frustrating because often I was in a position of being responsible for the program without the commensurate authority. Also, I was in a position of being liaison person between the hospital administrator and the psychiatrist, and *that's* a real dilemma. However, the program withstood its growing pains.

Question:

Was there a job description set us for you when you changed positions and went to the guidance clinic or did you negotiate for your role as it emerged from the community?

Miss Carlton:

I negotiated with the director when he offered me the change to work there, since he knew what I was doing in the community. The philosophy of the clinic is still quite traditional. However, the expectation was met that I would be involved in the community since I was asked if I would make "home visits." I've been allowed to move out into the community. Subsequently, other professionals gradually ventured into the community. Because of my interest and experience in developing programs, the director has recently asked me to lead a group to evaluate the ongoing programs and develop some new ones. I believe there is an advantage to not having a job description in these pioneering roles. It offers an opportunity for the nurse to set her own pace, depending on the climate or situation. In retrospect, I think I moved too quickly in the hospital. When I have patients in the hospital, I follow them and provide consultation as needed.

Comment:

I'd like to respond to how quickly you moved. In my community we started out with consultation and education, and involved the community in the planning of the center over a period of ten years. The psychiatric nursing specialist went into the hospital once a month, for 7 to 8 years of work, involving all of the nursing staff in the process. The amount of time spent there increased as the interest increased. The people who were most interested in mental health nursing formed a group and moved into the community mental health unit when it was opened. We still have inservice education for all the supervisors in the general hospital and also rotate our staff into the medical and surgical unit of the hospital so that there is a lot of sharing.

Comment:

We had that battle but we took another road. Nursing administration wanted to pull the psychiatric nurse into the general hospital and pull the psychiatric emergency room nurses into the general hospital emergency room. We said "No, we can't run a psychiatric unit that way."

Mrs. Carlton:

Our philosophy is different. Our approach is to help the caretakers in the community and to help the people who have problems in every area of the community. For instance, there are people on the medical and surgical units who need psychiatric nursing care, and the nurses there need to work with them.

Comment:

Your experience parallels mine. I'm presently in a squeeze play with one administration responsible for part of the service and another administration for the rest of it. You speak of how valuable just one nurse can be. A nurse can develop programs by bringing to bear her perceptions of problems and modes of meeting those problems. She may facilitate the services of these programs either directly or through consultation.

One of the things we need to be sensitive about is, can we realistically appraise what it is we can change and what we cannot change? As leaders, we have to confront people with the change-agent role and some of the consequences of that role.

Comment:

First, in regard to change, change is something that has to be really implemented from within the system and the change-agent can bring pressure to bear but the ultimate responsibility for the change must be assumed by the people involved in the system. This means that the people who bring the pressure to bear and get things stirred up should be different from the people who follow through, because the change-agent becomes the target of a lot of anger. For progress to take place, it is necessary for us to consider moving in, giving it everything we have, and then moving out at the appropriate time.

Comment:

I feel many more nurses are in a position to bring about change but they do not recognize negotiable items in regard to their function. Moreover, I think we deny our interest in liking power. We must have power in order to be self determining in terms of our role. And, our effectiveness is diluted when we assume responsibility without the authority to implement our ideas.

Comment:

I think the horrible struggle that exists between nursing and medicine is based on the belief that the doctor feels that the nurse wants to take his medical responsibility and authority away from him. I think the struggle will be over when we have convinced the doctors it's not the medical authority we want but the *rational* authority that comes from knowledge and skill.

Comment:

I have the responsibility for caring for patients but I don't have the power to make decisions regarding the patient. For example, I may make ten decisions about what my patient needs but I have no power to get things for them or have things carried out. I see an individual client or a family, but I can't have him admitted to the hospital, or decide on what type of treatment he needs, or discharge him, when I think it is important to do so.

Comment:

I function in a rigid, bureaucratic structure where I feel powerless. Yet, I'm supposed to be going out into the community and working with people who also feel powerless. They are really subject to the same kind of force. Maybe it has a different form, but basically, I think there are certain common elements operating in both our situations. I think I have to learn how to be more powerful in my setting that I can help people who have similar kinds of problems. I personally feel that nurses ought to be good for that kind of work because we have been second-class citizens. I would be interested in how others feel about feeling powerless—how others operate to become powerful and to help other people to become more powerful.

Comments:

What you're experiencing is related to the powerlessness of being a nurse. We oftentimes feel a sense of isolation from not only the social system we work in, but from the larger system of nursing. We frequently are unable to share in decision-making. Moreover, community mental health nursing is a new, uncharted area, and that creates anxiety. Perhaps what we're doing at this conference will give us some security and that, in turn, will give us some power.

If you expected to completely change the world which, it seems, some people are trying to do, you would have always ended up feeling helpless because it is something you just can not do.

I'm not sure where that powerlessness is coming from. I mean, have we decided that we're powerless so that we don't even look at possible ways of getting into the social political system? Or is it something else?

We need to be much more "with it" as far as our social systems theory and change theory is concerned. How do we analyze the situation? How do we intervene—particularly within the political structure—whether the political structure is part of an institution or whether it is the larger political structure out in the community.

Nurses have trouble understanding power and influence. We need to know that you get power because you have something the other person needs and wants, and it's not always information or education—initially, at least. You need a good understanding of what you have to trade and then later allow your education, knowledge, and skills to become the power exchange.

I've had to struggle with the issue of power over and over again. For example, I had an adolescent drug addict one night who needed to be admitted. I recognize that many professionals do not want to work with drug addicts—it's so unsuccessful. The addict is usually black, usually from lower income, nearly always from the ghetto and—there are always problems. At the same time, when someone needs to be admitted, I go ahead and admit him. If the administration is going to yell, you know that happens, I go to the director of nursing. I've had to put my job on the line in terms of what I'm going to demand to be done. You go to who's over you and if you're a good person, you make those demands. I don't have any degrees but I get the kind of support I need. I've made mistakes, but so have the doctors. I repeat, it does mean putting your job on the line sometimes, but it also means you define how much you're willing to do with that job—how important it is to you to resolve differences that affect clients.

You have to determine what is needed and get out there and do it. You take responsibility instead of asking permission. We were told we couldn't take nurse aides out in the community. We got together and worked up our inservice program. We started teaching the nurse aides what we both wanted and took them out on home visits with us and it was done. There was no valid objection then, because there were no grounds. It was happening, and they were supervised, and they were valuable in many ways that professionals could not have been.

Comment:

I can add to that. I just began, but I'm sure it's going to work. We have this merger of three hospitals and we're looking around now to see what services we're going to discontinue, what services we're going to maintain, and what new services we're going to include. I've drawn up 34 suggestions, and I've documented how they can be accomplished, and I've sent them to the administrator. I think you have to take the initiative and get the ball rolling. Just asset yourself. Be there first, and be prepared to identify what needs to be done, why it needs to be done, and how it can be done. You think fast, you talk loudly, and you win.

Comment:

Power also comes from the community. We involved paraprofessionals in our system but were unable to change the system from within to give them mobility and commensurate salaries. We took the problem to the community, resulting in the introduction of a whole new series of mental health workers, with higher salaries, and with a chance for upward mobility. The new system was introduced and pushed through the legislature through the power of the community. We had tried, and tried, and tried, and we couldn't work with bureaucracy. But, with the power from the community, we succeeded.

Comment:

In my state, the state nurses' association exerted influence in defining what psychiatric nurses can do. We did not ask the medical community what we could do. We just said, "We are the people who define psychiatric nursing practice in this state."

Comment:

Nurses need to organize committees to define appropriate practice. In addition, these committees, or action groups, ought to deal with the experiences patients are exposed to, or have to put up with, and they are often inhumane. We get ourselves appointed to various governor's commissions that do influence what happens. We work through our state legislators. We ask them to state their position on legislation which affects us and our clients. We let them know that we have a certain number of voters in their district and that we are watching their decisions and will act accordingly at election time.

Comment:

People are referring to power and how we can get it and use it in several ways. Talking from my own experience in the community mental health area, I was struck by the power and the *power potential* and I wonder how we could use this in an effective way in working with people, in helping communities, and in overall county planning, to bring about relevant services? I hope we will focus on power more than powerlessness. I really feel we have a great deal of power when we choose to use it. Moreover, we are willing to share power which is really the critical issue. Nurses are crusaders and innovators in our communities. We *are* change-agents.

Part Two
Theoretical
Explorations

THEORETICAL EXPLORATIONS

Theoretical explorations are necessary for the nurse's assessment and maintenance of, or intervention in, the various interacting mental health processes and
systems. These chapters are written by three experts* in the field of mental
health. The need for this second part was established by the conferees during the
three-day conference when they advanced the following:

> As a change agent, the community mental health nurse possesses a
> theoretical knowledge and understanding of social systems, power, and
> change. This enhances the nurse's ability to become involved with social
> issues, social action, and social change in order to institute and
> implement preventive programs relevant to individuals, families, and the
> community.

Conferees reported that community mental health nurses, as well as other
community mental health personnel, learn about social systems, power, and
change primarily through the work situation, which often is too little and too
late.

Conferees recognized that in part, this inadequacy resulted from a failure of
social scientists to generate knowledge about social systems in a form meaningful
and useful to practitioners. Conferees agreed that this knowledge is one of the
prerequisites for nursing practice to have relevance to the needs of clients and
the community.

---

*Grayce L. Sills, Ph.D., R. N. Graduate School of Nursing, Program in Nursing, Ohio State
University, Columbus, Ohio. Anita Werner O'Toole, Ph.D., R. N. Associate Professor,
School of Nursing, Case Western Reserve University, Cleveland, Ohio. Eugene B. Nadler,
Ph.D. Social Scientist, Maimonides Comprehensive Community Mental Health Center,
Brooklyn, New York.

Social Systems and Mental Health Services

GRAYCE SILLS, R.N., PH.D

INTRODUCTION

There is much in the social science literature about the systems of arrangements that humans have evolved over time to attempt to solve basic human problems.[1,2] More recently some social system theorists have attempted to meld their work with that of the general systems theorists.[3,4] Such theoretical explanations offer much to a conceptualization of complex sets of functional components in interaction. Since this book focuses on mental health and mental illness the effort in this chapter will be to examine the sets of components and their interactions vis-a-vis the system of services for care and prevention of mental illness.

THE CONCEPTUAL FRAMEWORK

This chapter will outline a conceptual framework to describe and explain the pathways to care organizations. The discussion and presentation of the framework can be divided into four parts. The first part outlines a general overview for the pathways to the care system. The second part deals with the process of social control and its relevance for the pathways to care services. The third dimension discussed is that of the definition and decision-making process. The fourth and final part of the framework elaborates the movement into and out of the services for care of the mentally ill. Each part will be discussed separately, and literature will be cited to document the relevance of the proposed framework to important work in the field.

The General Overview

The behavioral phenomena that have come to be designated as mental illness are socially recognized as existing in varying degrees of severity, and requiring varying responses from society. The societal designations and corresponding societal responses constitute a flow-model for the processes, and work to maintain the balance between the demand for services generated by the gradient definitions of mental illness and the variety of organizational responses which constitute the supply of services.

Figure 1 diagrams the general framework. Society is seen as providing both the consumers and purveyors of the services in the mental illness care system. Entry into the system is regulated by the process of social control. The sub-set of persons defined as mentally ill, about whom a decision has been made to enter them into the services system, becomes eligible for a wide range of services. These services are provided by both the public and private sectors of society.

THE PROCESS OF SOCIAL CONTROL. The process of social control operates to define the entrants to the services, and the norms and values of society provide the matrix around which social life is organized. Values relate to standards of desirability, and norms regulate conduct. Norms prescribe and proscribe certain kinds of actions by various actors in different situations, and cultural norms are widely shared by individuals in society. One way to know norms is by inference. In the case of mental illness, it can be said that persons defined as mentally ill reflect nonconformity to the shared norms of behavior. Thus society regulates the behavior of the members by sanctioning that behavior according to standards set and shared.

In industrial and urban societies many sets of norms are formalized. Laws have been written to codify procedures used to deal with mental illness, and the legal system is one means of social control in the mental illness services system. The law helps to define the conditions under which entrants to the mental illness system are deprived of certain civil rights and liberties. The mental illness services system represents one of the major articulating points in this society for the institutions of medicine and law.[5]

THE DEFINERS OF MENTAL ILLNESS. The definers of mental illness come from several sources. There are three major categories of definers: the societally legitimated mental health professionals, the legally empowered societal agents, those who represent "significant others" to the protagonist, and the "self."

THE PROFESSIONAL DEFINERS. The professional mental illness definers constitute those in our society who have been called the "paid

I. THE POPULATION   II. THE DEFINING PROCESS   III. SOCIETAL RESPONSES   IV. MENTAL ILLNESS
                         SOCIAL CONTROL   SERVICES FOR CARE

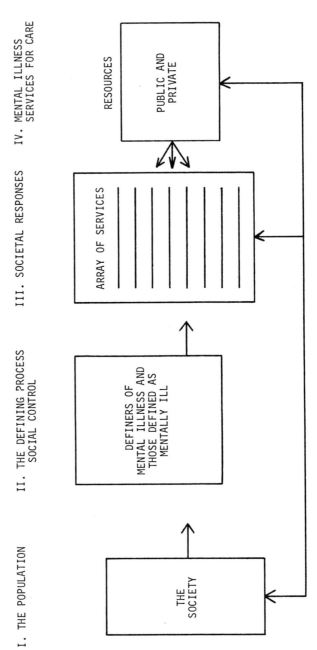

Fig. 1. Conceptual framework for the organization of health care for the mentally ill.

altruists."* This group is made up of physicians, nurses, psychologists, and social workers. The persons in these professional groups probably now number 754,000–305,000 physicians, 621,000 nurses, 125,000 social workers, and 18,000 psychologists.[6] However, only a portion of each of these groups is likely to be engaged in the defining process. In the physician group, 92,000 general practitioners and 20,000 psychiatrists would constitute the primary defining group. Of the 600,000 nurses there are 18,010 who work in mental health establishments and 41,254 in public health nursing. Hence, there are roughly 60,000 nurses who have active potential as mental illness definers. Of the 125,000 social workers, 11,200 are working in psychiatric settings. More than any other group, almost all social workers could be categorized as primary definers of mental illness. Of the group of psychologists about 6,000 are in clinical psychology, and thus would be apt to be active in the defining process. This brings the total number of primary definers to 189,000.[7] Together with the police, this group might aptly be called the "gatekeepers" to the mental illness services system.**

Secondary definers would be physicians, nurses, and psychologists who work in schools and industry, plus school teachers and the clergy. In the volume, *The Churches and Mental Health*, McCann reports that while more than one-third of all counseling problems seen by the clergy are estimated to be of serious psychiatric dimensions, only one-tenth of them are ever referred to psychiatric resources.[8]

All together, the secondary definers constitute an unknown number of persons who may have (but often do not have), a significant import on the entrance of persons into the mental health services system. It is likely that they serve as a kind of pre-screening and refer to the "professional help-givers" for definition, rather than making the definition directly.

THE LEGAL DEFINERS. The law which is so intimately bound to the mental illness system in this country serves as the protector of society and the individual. The law and its agents—the courts, the police, and health officials—serve as major gatekeepers for entrance to the mental illness care services.

The law provides the framework in which the legal definers do their work, and generally assumes both a medical and a moral stance. Typically, the individual is to be confined in a hospital when he is endangering lives or property. Just as is true in criminal law, the law as it pertains to mental disability primarily serves those whose behavior is officially noticed. It is usually the enforcers of the law, police, deputy sheriffs, peace officers, and so on, who have the greatest opportunity for defining a person as mentally ill.

*I am indebted to Dr. Harold Pepinsky, Professor of Psychology, The Ohio State University, for this felicitous phrase. I do not know if it is original with him.

**This graphic expression was brought to our attention in an unpublished paper by Irwin Deutscher, "The Gatekeeper in Public Housing," read at the annual meeting of the Eastern Sociological Society, April 1, 1961.

Such agents have the authority to effect temporary emergency confinement in all but 12 of the 50 states. Confinement usually takes place in a state or county mental hospital, but in a few states, jail is sometimes used. Almost all involuntary hospitalization for mental illness involves the use of legal enforcers. According to Schwartz, "A court officer or a policeman is the patient's frequent escort, and often the patient is unaccompanied by friends or family."[9] Such circumstances would seem to have a profound bearing on the "defining process" as well as the potential outcomes for a person as he moves through the mental illness system.

"CLOSE OTHERS" AS DEFINERS. The legal system and the family system support the idea that close relatives and close friends are expected to be involved in the process of making the definition of mental illness. The typical language of the law is "friend, relative, spouse, guardian, or health officer."[10] Mechanic emphasizes that "community members," *not* professional personnel, are the initial definers.[11] The importance of the family and others to the defining process is further underscored in this quote from Thomas Schaff about those cases in which the family or close others initiated hospitalization: "These cases are pretty *automatic*. If the patient's own family wants to get rid of him you know there is something wrong."[12]

SELF AS DEFINER. Logically it would seem that all who voluntarily admit themselves to clinics, hospitals, or other facilities, are in fact making the initial definition for themselves. Apparently what is sought by these "self-definers" is validation that the definition is a tenable one. When self is the initial definer it seem likely there has been some prior involvement in the decision making by "close others."

THE SOCIETAL RESOURCES. Society invests certain of its resources to provide the array of services available to the person defined as mentally ill. The resources have their source in the private or public sectors of the society. It is a historical fact that the cost for the care of mental illness has been largely borne by the public sector. Almshouses usually contained a section for the "lunaticks." Later the States made provision for the care and confinement of the mentally ill. Until the early 1950's, the Federal government continued the stance adopted by President Franklin Pierce in 1854 when he vetoed the "12,225,000 Acre Bill" which would have given the states additional financial support for care programs for the mentally ill. President Pierce held that "Congress did not have this power to usurp State's rights—even in defense of human rights." It was almost a century later that the Federal government began financial participation with the states in the provision of services.[13]

THE ARRAY OF SERVICES

The array of services for the mentally ill can be classified in two categories—outpatient services and inpatient services. These may be sub-classified by the type of control—public or private.

1. OUTPATIENT SERVICES.– In the wake of the Joint Commission report, *Action for Mental Health*, outpatient services expanded more rapidly than any other category of service. Typically the outpatient services are organized around the clinic model. The professional experts occupy offices in a structure, often attached to a general hospital, and the patient brings himself to the source of the service. In the past decade there has been considerable development of clinics unattached to a hospital. These facilities more often are found in smaller cities and towns. Some clinics are established in conjunction with the courts, usually juvenile courts. More clinics seem to be multipurpose organizations. In a broad sense, their stated purpose is the prevention of mental illness. Given the imprecise criteria about what behavior should be defined as mental illness, is it not surprising that clinics are less than precise in stating organizational objectives.

Many outpatient services apparently are becoming "gatekeepers" for the inpatient hospital. A number of patients to the clinic are referred by other community agencies. A large percentage of those who present themselves to clinics are self or family referred.

There seems to be two major functions, or organizational objectives, of the clinic as a type of outpatient service, validation services, and treatment services. The validation function of a clinic is provided in the form of judgments about a person's health status that will be widely accepted by third parties and is a major reason for referral to the clinics from other agencies. This validation role is illustrated in this citation from Fuchs:

> *Consider the following situation: a person is thought to be acting peculiar, he has various problems which seem to be worrying him. He complains and looks for sympathy from family, friends, neighbors and co-workers. He may seek to be relieved from certain responsibilities or to be excused from certain tasks. Doubts may arise in the minds of persons around him. Questions may be asked. Is he really ill? Is he doing all that he can to get well? A visit, or a series of visits to a clinic or a physician may be indicated. The patient may not have the slightest hope that these visits will help his health, and, indeed he may be correct. Nevertheless, the service rendered by the clinic cannot be said to result in no output. The visit to the clinic or physician is a socially or culturally necessary act. The examination, the diagnosis, and the prognosis are desired by the patient and the agency to provide confirmation to those who have doubts about him. Only the professional judgment can still the doubts and answer the questions.*[14]

The second major function is direct care services. The individual may be accepted as an active case and his treatment may include individual and group psychotherapy, medication, occupational therapy, sometimes electroshock therapy, and occasionally some form of ambulatory insulin therapy. Any one or a combination of several of the above may constitute the therapeutic modality for the direct care service function of the clinic.

Another organizational objective may be operative in the workings of the outpatient clinic, and that is the delivery of mental health services to the community. In this instance the community is conceptualized at the "patient." Treatment is delivered by educating key professional groups in mental health concepts—teachers, nurses, general medical practitioners, clergymen, and others. Consultation for mental health problems is offered to established social welfare agencies, and the "lay" population (P.T.A. groups, home-study clubs, service clubs, and voluntary organizations).

There are other organizations related to outpatient services. In most communities there is usually a group of health and welfare organizations having a direct or indirect relationship to mental illness care services. *Directly*, the function may be counseling for the purpose of prevention of mental illness, for example, some family and children's agencies. *Indirectly*, the function may be prevention through education, for example, the educational programs of a mental health association. The number and kinds of these health and welfare agencies in a given community will likely affect the rate and direction of the flow into the mental illness services system.

Persons in help-giving occupations who operate entrepreneurially represent part of the outpatient services provided by society. This category would include psychiatrists, psychoanalysts, nonmedical psychotherapists (usually clinical psychologists), and perhaps an occasional psychiatric nurse or psychiatric social worker practicing independently. Marginal to the above group of more or less "legitimate" helpgivers are the palm readers, fortune tellers, consulting astrologists, soothsayers, spiritualistic mediums, and others of this genre. Both types of entrepreneurs have as their chief purpose the giving of help to persons who are troubled—for a fee. In other words, they provide outpatient services for those who can afford them. The former, because they are more legitimate, have more ties to the established mental illness services system. The latter operate in a largely marginal position with regard to the society as a whole and seldom have a direct point of articulation with the mental illness care services. This marginal group of paid help-givers has been largely unexplored in the social science literature. In a speculative way one might guess that some of these practitioners in a sense, may be highly skilled "help-givers."

Single service organizations sometimes develop in a community to take care of one aspect of the spectrum of mental illness. The various suicide prevention services, Alcoholics Anonymous, Synanon, Parents Without Partners, and Senior Citizens are representative of this type of group. Their relationship to the mental illness system is likely to be partially determined by the degree to which the organization is professionally controlled. Some of this effort seems to have as an ostensible purpose the reduction of "stigma." The group and the concern of the group is a deviant concern, but the clustering together of "we are all of a kind" seems to provide a kind of support for persons who possess a "stigmatized self."[15] Many people are likely to be extruded from these service groups because they fail to act in a sufficiently normative manner for the "deviant" group. This type of group also can serve as a catchment for products of the inpatient services.

Borderline to outpatient and inpatient services is a group of services offered by agencies in the community, usually with the general aim of preventing the need for full-time hospitalization. Such services may include a "home" for alcoholics, and day or night care in mental hospitals.

Aftercare Services

Aftercare services for the mentally ill vary widely in the nature and kinds of services provided. All aftercare services are explicitly expected to help the former patient re-establish himself in the community, but the high relapse or readmission rate in mental illness suggests that perhaps in no other area of deviancy is this feat so difficult to accomplish.

The most common form of aftercare is the outpatient clinic. The hospital is obliged morally, and often legally, to "guarantee" that the ex-patient will not be "turned loose" in the community. One needs only to read a newpaper account of a crime involving a personal offense committed by an ex-patient or a patient on leave from a mental hospital, to assess the very serious nature of the bargain which hospitals and community strike with one another. Thus the aftercare clinic characteristically "keeps an eye on" the ex-patient. Medication, particularly the psychotropic drugs, perhaps some psychotherapy, and always the assistance of the social worker, constitute the staples of the aftercare clinic. The social worker is essential, either to assist in the job placement or to help in negotiation of the bureaucratic maze to secure the financial assistance necessary if a job is not available, feasible or tenable.[16]

Other types of aftercare services are foster homes and nursing homes whereby the mentally ill patient can, in effect, be transferred to a different care setting. Both types of facilities seem to be used most often in planning for the elderly and the chronic patient, and thus are aftercare services in a very limited sense.

Halfway houses—temporary homes to bridge the gap between hospital and community—represent another form of aftercare services. In American society it is "good" to work. Work establishes a place in society for a person. Job and work training programs are important. Thus sheltered workshops and vocation rehabilitation centers are important in aftercare services.

The ex-patient club is an interesting, if not widespread, type of aftercare program. These "therapeutic clubs" are formed by ex-patients to facilitate social adjustment. Perhaps the best known of these is Fountain House in New York City. Fountain House officials claim that ex-patients who avail themselves of this service have a return rate (to the hospital) of 3.6 percent compared to an average, national return rate of about 25 percent.[17] Generally, ex-mental patient clubs have not become widespread, compared to colostomy clubs, "the lost chords," and others.

The eventual goal of the aftercare services is to facilitate the ex-patient's re-entry into the community and to maintain that entry once it has been established. Most reports suggest that this successful ending is not often attained. More recently the effect has seemed to be more like a revolving door to the community than a one-way exit from the hospital. Indeed, it may be that in unintended ways, the aftercare system perpetuates the return flow.

Inpatient Services

Inpatient care is provided in a variety of organizational settings. The historic fact of the Federal government's abdication of the responsibility for the care of the mentally ill to the states in American society has resulted in the state mental hospital becoming the largest single type or organizational response to mental illness.[18] Inpatient psychiatric facilities are provided also by the Veterans Administration, voluntary non-profit hospitals, and proprietary hospitals.

The state mental hospital, of course, provides care for most of the inpatient mentally ill. One distinguishing feature of the typical state mental hospital is its large size. Of the 337 longterm, non-Federal psychiatric hospitals, 276 have 500 beds or over. Better than 80 percent of these hospitals are large hospitals; a few reach a magnitude of 18 thousand beds. Other, salient characteristics of the typical state mental hospital are low personnel-patient ratios, low expenditure rate per patient per day, and low patient turnover.

The private inpatient care sector provides services by units in short-term, nongovernmental hospitals, and proprietary psychiatric hospitals. In 1966, 12.4 percent of the short-term, nongovernmental hospitals had inpatient psychiatric facilities. All the statistics for this discussion have been taken from the source cited in reference 18. It is well to remember that the data include "marginal" facilities to the mental illness system. That is, special hospitals for addiction, alcohol, and narcotics, chiefly; hospitals serving the mentally retarded are also included. Thus the system seems larger in scope than it may actually be, yet the marginal facilities probably do enter into the ebb and flow of the system and it seems wise to count them in.

SOCIAL CONTROL AND MENTAL ILLNESS

When society is reviewed in a problem-solving perspective, two problems are of concern. First, the problem of adaptation to man's biosocial nature, resulting in the development of societal arrangements for the care of illness; second, the problem of adaptation to collective living must be considered. Rules, therefore, are elaborated to cover the gamut of human relations. The way in which a society decides to solve these problems will derive in part from the values shared by society at large. The development of norms to regulate the conduct of society, reflects in part the values of the society, but also may contradict those values. In regard to mental illness, a complex set of norms has evolved to guide the process of social control; a complex set or organizational arrangements also has been developed to care for the mentally ill. These norms and arrangements can be expected to vary with age, sex, marital status, sub-cultures, rural-urban residence, and a host of other factors. However, there seems to be several common features in the overall process of social control. First, the norms typically carry both official and unofficial sanctions; second, the arrangements for care are simple or complex, depending on the structure of the community—particularly the mental health manpower resources. Figure 2 diagrams the interconnections of these complex features of the process of social control in mental illness.

Values

The dominant values in this society are typically those of the middle class. Davis recognized the significance of this fact in relations to the mental hygiene movement, and specifically notes the moral-scientific dilemma:

> *Mental hygiene cannot combine the prestige of science with the prestige of the mores, for science and then mores unavoidably conflict, and the point where they most readily conflict is precisely where "mental," i.e., social phenomena, are concerned.*[19]

Almost 20 years later, John Seeley argued that since the Industrial Revolution the market has come to be the dominant institution, and there has been a decline in the mystical organizing qualities of the family, the church, and the guild. Thus no one institution firmly proclaims what is the good life, what is the order of the virtues, and so on. This has created a power vacuum and the mental health movement has been drawn into this vacuum. Seeley credits the mental health movement with making society aware of the inner life of man and its relation to his external life. According to Seeley, the mental health movement has become an arbiter between scientific knowledge and lay utilization of that knowledge:

> *What seems to be emerging is a situation in which laymen—ordinary men and women—in their everyday activites are coming to use a new body of knowledge and techniques of analysis with reference to themselves and to one another. The importance of this may not be immediately evident, but the effect is almost as though another dimension (and another complication) had been added to life.*

He also strikes a note of alarm:

> *The mental health movement is underway—no one can alter that broad sweep of events, but the moral responsibility of the mental health movement is clear—proximate and remote consequences of the values and ideas promoted must be subjected to close and continuing research, for to do otherwise is to invite disaster.*[20]

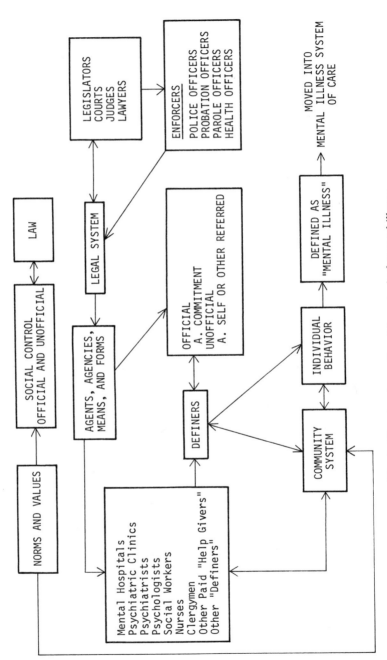

Fig. 2. The structure of social control of mental illness.

Empirical support for both the Davis and Seeley positions is found in a content analysis study of mental health pamphlets. The conclusion reached was that the middle-class prototype and the mental health prototype in many respects are equivalent. The authors of one study say that with Davis, they conclude that the mental health movement is "unwittingly propagating a middle-class ethic under the guise of science."[21] This study also suggests that the class bias in the mental health movement, while it purports to foster individual integration to the extent that it supports middle-class social organization, may in effect be producing that which it intends to combat.

Norms

The majority of persons trained in mental health professions come from middle-class backgrounds, which suggests that the mental health professions share the middle-class bias. This in turn influences both legal and medical aspects of social control to the mental illness services system. Even in these groups, however, there is lack of consensus about what the norms should be. For example in the survey of the literature done by Marie Jahoda for the Joint Commission on Mental Illness and Health, she concludes that there is no standard, all-purpose definition of mental health. In fact, different people have different standards and these vary widely. In the last chapter of the Jahoda statement, the psychiatric clinician Dr. Walter Barton expresses a viewpoint wherein the absence of mental illness is the key: "If they are not sick, they are well."[22]

The establishment of unofficial norms are rooted in the biases of the middle-class ethic. The unofficial system of social control seems to have its primary source in the better educated, the mental health professionals, and other assorted helping professions. These groups claim to have the expertise to make the mental illness definition and their claim is usually honored. In a newspaper item on page 11 in the *Columbus Citizen-Journal* of September 19, 1968, a psychiatrist speaking to a group of clergymen is quoted as saying, ". . . ministers could be helpful in 'propagandizing' the principles governing normal interaction among families. By acquainting people with the norms it would be easier for them to recognize departures and thus recognize problems early before they become serious." Studies tend to document the use of very broad norms by professional help providers. Apparently, the more education a person has, the broader the criteria become.[23] One study finds that when presented with six case histories, psychiatrists tended to define mentally ill to non-mentally ill in the ratio of 9:1. The average ratio for the laymen was 1:2. The lay criteria used as a guide for decisions seem to be based on the "raving maniac" stereotype. Cumming and Cumming assert that for the layman anything less than that stereotype is assessed as "it's just a quirk–a little nervousness–personality traits–nothing serious."[24] Part of the professionals' criteria is that early recognition of symptoms can prevent severe consequences, and although that criteria has not been well documented, it continues to be used. In fact, it continues to be used despite some evidence to the contrary.[25] Nevertheless, it seems a valid assumption elsewhere in the sphere of medicine, and this may be the basis for its continued use by the mental health professions. Nothing in recent history suggests that the gap in views between the professionals and the laity is narrowing. Both the Seeley and the Cummings' have documented the sad fate of mental health education efforts at the community level.[26,27]

The end result of the process of social control is that the person sanctioned by whatever norms is moved into the system of mental illness care services. Central to understanding this movement is knowledge about the defining-decision-making process. We now turn to that discussion.

THE DEFINING-DECISION-MAKING PROCESS

It is necessary logically, to conceptualize the defining process as a decision-making process. For example, to *label* a given behavioral event "sick" serves only to name it, or to categorize it with a similar class of events. But to *define* a behavioral event as "sick" is to make a decision about meaning. To give an event meaning is to imbue it with past, present, and future significance for both the definer and the defined. Giving meaning is a dynamic act which purports a future consequence for both the definer and the defined. Thus a course of action is prescribed in which the protagonist is moved into the mental illness services system.[27] It is well to note here Goffman's point about how comfortable the social sciences have become in using the term, "deviant." He infers that it may be serving social science as the iatrogenic disorders serve medicine, to give social scientists more work to do. Figure 3 diagrams the possibilities for varying patterns of definition-decision-making as a part of social control.

Scheff, in his explanation of stable mental illness as a residual deviance, states as his final causal hypothesis: "Among residual rule breakers, labeling is the most important cause of careers of residual deviance."[28] There is agreement that labeling is of crucial importance to careers of residual deviance, and while labeling may be sufficient to explain "stable mental illness," it does not seem sufficient to explain entrance into the mental illness services system. In the present view it is not the rule-breaking that is crucial, but the sanctioned official or unofficial definitional process, the process which results in moving the person into mental illness care services.

> The likelihood that residual rule-breaking in itself will not lead to labeling as a deviant draws attention to the central significance of the contingencies which influence the direction and intensity of the societal reaction. One of the urgent conceptual tasks for a sociological theory of deviant behavior is the development of a precise and widely applicable set of such contingencies. The classification that is offered here is only a crude first step in this direction.

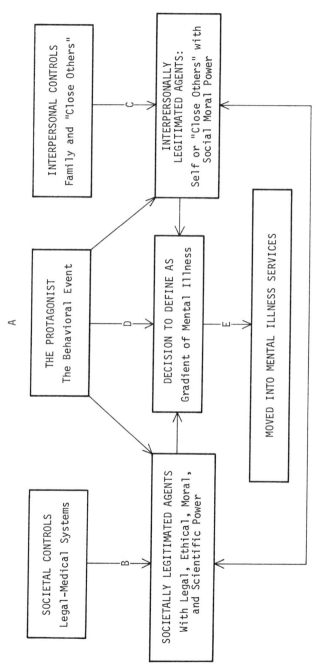

Fig. 3. The definition-decision-making process.

199

Although there are a wide variety of contingencies which lead to labeling they can be simply classified in terms of the nature of the rule-breaking, the person who breaks the rules, and the community in which the rule-breaking occurs. Other things being equal, the severity of the societal reaction is a function of, first, the degree, amount and visibility of the rule breaking; second, the power of the rule-breaker, and the social distance between him and the agents of social control; and finally, the tolerance level of the community, and the availability in the culture of the community of alternative nondeviant roles. Particularly crucial for future research is the importance of the first two contingencies (the amount and degree of rule-breaking), which are characteristics of the rule-breaker, relative to the remaining five contingencies, which are characteristics of the social system. To the extent that these five factors are found empirically to be independent determinants of labeling and denial, the status of the mental patient can be considered a partly ascribed rather than a completely achieved status. The dynamics of treated mental illness could then be profitably studied quite apart from the individual dynamics of mental disorder by focusing on social systemic contingencies.[29]

The position taken in this chapter of the mental illness services system differs somewhat from Scheff's. This framework assumes a mental illness services system in the society with differential access based on a number of factors. It further speaks to a broader spectrum of deviance, whereas Scheff confines his explanation to residual rule-breaking and residual deviance. Becker advises that it is fallacious to assume that all who have broken a rule will be labeled deviant, or that all who are labeled deviant have in fact broken a rule.[30]

The view taken here is not a psychiatric one but rather a sociological one. A view which suggests that when a person is defined in such a way that the definition leads to a decision for entrance into the mental illness services for care, a significant alteration has been made in that person's social life. Hence, more than labeling is involved in the process, though labeling may be a part of it.

PATTERNS OF DEFINITION–DECISION-MAKING

Figure 3 suggests that different patterns may develop in the relationships among the persons in categories A, B, and C. The power referred to in B and C can be distinguished by the source of the legitimation of the power: that is, B is impersonal power and the source of legitimation is in the social structure. C is personal power and the source of legitimation is in the interpersonal structure. It is where A, B and C meet at point D to make a decision about A that the "personal troubles of milieu and the public issues of social structure" converge. Until this time, what has been a trouble has been a private matter and according to Mills it now becomes an issue " . . . which often involves a crisis in institutional relationships."[31] Several possible patterns or pathways are indicated by the conceptual framework.

The Others-Official Pattern

The A, B, D, E pattern can be referred to as an "others-official" pattern. It is likely to occur when there is a poverty of relationships in C. This pathway is a most typical one for entry to the state mental hospital. The empirical studies which have findings that relate high rates of mental illness to categories of persons in "disengaged" statuses—the aged, widowed, formerly married but not now married, and so on—document this pattern.*

The Others-Unofficial Pattern

The "others-unofficial" the A, C, D, E pattern, acknowledges power differentials within networks of interpersonal relationships. It further suggests that there is a possibility of entrance into the mental illness system without reference to the official agents of·control in the social system. It is likely the less status "self" has in reference to the "significant other" the more likely is the "other" to be the prime definer. Hence, one would expect parents to be able to define their young children, but adult children to be able to define their elderly parents.

The "others-unofficial" pattern is vulnerable and often has to have *post facto* validation for the definition to hold. Thus a variant pattern develops. Here the self or close others ask the societal agents to validate the definition and ratify the decision. Goffman has referred to their kind of pattern from the point of view of the protagonist as the "betrayal funnel."[32] Scheff, in one study, came to the conclusion that in metropolitan areas the legal and medical decision-making was largely ceremonial—that the crucial decisions had already been made by the relatives or others who brought the cases to court.[33] Kutner further documents the almost automatic ratification of the definition, and the decision already made by lay persons.[34]

Complementing these studies is an investigation by Wenger, who asked the question: What happens if the protagonist is represented by legal counsel at the ratification hearing? Wenger calls the group he studied "pre-patients." In the present conceptual framework they would be seen as having already entered the services system, and the hearing would be for the purpose of ratifying a decision already made. Hence, the commitment hearing would determine if the definition

*All of these studies cannot be cited. However, for example, see: Srole, et al. *Mental Health in the Metropolis*, New York, Basic Books, Inc., 1959; Lowenthal, M.F., Social isolation and mental illness in old age, Amer. Sociol. Rev. 29:54-70, Feb. 1964. Tangentially, though they deal with pathways out of the system, the work of Dinitz, et al, Psychiatric and social attributes as predictors of case outcome in mental hospitalization, *Social Problems*, 8:322-328, Spring, 1961, is relevant for this formulation, inasmuch as the process of staying out of the hospital is likely to be influenced by the same variables as those which determine how the patient got in in the first place.

is to hold. As Scheff and Kutner have noted, this process is usually perfunctory. Wenger showed the presence of legal counsel and the release from a commitment hearing to be highly correlated—.942. It would seem that the agents of the legal system, acting in behalf of the protagonist, can affect the medical decision. Thus, the original decision, made either in B or C, while usually ratified by agents of B, is subject to reversal—but seldom is, as Wenger further reports. Of 81 patients who were observed, 65 were committed; 61 of these were without legal counsel.[35]

The "Self-Official" Pattern

The "self-official," pattern is represented in the A to D to B to E pathway. The protagonist makes his own definition and seeks validation for it by the societally-legitimated definers, receives it, and enters the services system. Goffman refers to this as the "dubious privilege of the upper middle class."[36] This route is often taken to the outpatient clinic, the private psychiatric hospital, or the psychoanalyst's couch and the psychotherapeutic hour. Generally, though not always, the gradient is defined in mild terms: emotional exhaustion, overwork and fatigue; excessive nervousness; and so on. Failure of this pattern to achieve what was desired by either the protagonist or the legitimator is discernible in several ways. First, the protagonist may withdraw, as happens so often in clinics. Second, the legitimator may decide a redefinition is needed in terms of the gradient factor. Here there are at least three alternatives: (1) the legitimator may directly act to redefine the situation in official terms; (2) he may seek to involve the persons in category C and persuade them to define the situation in such a way as to move the protagonist into another part of the services system; (3) the patient may be referred to another part of the services system.

A Variant Pattern

A variant pattern is initiated in organizations which deal in personal services. The personnel in schools and universities, the public health nursing service agencies and welfare agencies, are frequently charged with the responsibility of "case-finding." The "cases" in this context are usually referred to as psychiatric or mental health problems. Once found, the cases are usually referred to a mental health professional whose task it is to validate or refute the tentative definition made by the case-finder. If the definition is validated, the decision to act, that is to move the person into the mental illness services system, is usually then referred to the significant others.

The "Self-Unofficial" Pattern

The A, D, E pathway is seen in voluntary admissions to hospitals and self-referrals to clinics. Goffman argues for "willing and unwilling" as a useful distinction in terms of who comes to the mental hospital.[37] He suggests that only a relatively small group of "pre-patients" come into the hospital willingly. However, it seems possible that the self versus others distinction, operationally defined as voluntary versus official commitment to the hospital, can be a useful way of conceptualizing the differential degree of control the defined person may have over the situation in which he finds himself. The network of relationships in which the self operates are occasionally so impoverished that perhaps it makes little difference whether the patient is voluntarily or officially committed. But in most networks of interpersonal relationships it would seem likely that this contingency, voluntary versus official, would have many ramifications in that network of relationships.

This discussion has not exhausted all of the possible variations in the definitional-decision-making process. The focus instead has been on the major patterns. Social psychologists have demonstrated well the richness, variety and complexity of the patterns discussed here.[38, 39]

MOVEMENT INTO AND THROUGH
MENTAL ILLNESS SERVICES

Once the definition-decision has been made, movement follows into the system of services for care. Let us now turn to a discussion of the concomitants of that movement and some of the factors influencing entry and exit. Figure 4 diagrams the interconnections of the factors affecting the flow into the facilities for care, the types of facilities, and some factors which influence outcome.

Major factors which influence the definition-decision process are socio-demographic variables: age, sex, race, and marital status. The factor of self or others as definers, and the official or unofficial status of the definition will likely affect the mode of entry and the type of service. The kind and numbers of facilities for service in a community likely will be related to the total mental health manpower in the community, and this also affects the rate of entrance to care facilities.

The social characteristics of the community of residence (size and facilities for care) are important factors influencing rates and directions of pathways into the mental illness services system. Another factor is the economic resources of the individual. This would influence the point of entry into the services system. The degree of complexity of the mental illness services system is thought to be a factor influencing the flow through the services. The numbers of mental health professionals in the community of residence are an additional factor that might influence rates of entry into the system. Differential distribution of the various types of mental health manpower would be expected to influence rates and points of entry, for when there is a demand for services created by decisions made about gradients of mental illness, there is likely to be a response to the demand from the supply of agents and agencies, also gradiently defined. Uneven

A. DEFINITION-DECISION → B. FACILITIES FOR CARE → C. CONCOMITANTS AND OUTCOMES*

A. DEFINITION-DECISION

1. Self-official (ABDE)
2. Self-unofficial (ADE)
3. Others-official (ABDE)
4. Others-unofficial (ACDE)
5. Other variants

A. CONTINGENCIES

1. Socio-demographic factors
2. Self or others definition
3. Characteristics of the community of residence

B. FACILITIES FOR CARE

1. Private-outpatient
2. Public-outpatient
3. Private-inpatient
4. Public-inpatient a) Short term
                   b) Long term

B. CONTINGENCIES

1. Community resources
2. Community resource characteristics
3. Economic factors

C. CONCOMITANTS AND OUTCOMES*

	Stigma	Role Disruption	Movement Out
1.	0-+	0-+	Good
2.	+-++	0-+	Good-Fair
3.	+-++	+++-++++	Fair-Moderate
4a.	++-+++	+++-++++	Fair-Moderate
4b.	+++-++++	++++	Moderate-Poor

C. CONTINGENCIES

1. The combination of A and B contingencies

*The plus (+) signs represent crude assessments. Thus: + = slight; ++ = moderate; +++ = very great; ++++ = inevitable.

Fig. 4. Mental illness—the flow.

distribution of supply services will create problems of uneven access. Success in the sense that the services supplied are equal to the demand is often complicated by mismatched gradients. When this happens, negotiation is required, and the consumers and suppliers may bargain for other arrangements. Then decisions may be made to redefine the gradient in different terms which requires further movement within the system by the consumer.[40]

SUMMARY

What has been presented here represents an effort to conceptualize and describe the broad and complex system of services for care in mental illness. Such a conceptualization attempts to place that system within the larger societal system. Inasmuch as community mental health services do not exist in a vacuum nor do the clients of such services live in a vacuum, it seemed useful to view the arrangements for care and services in a wider perspective.

What community health workers need to do now is to test this and other models with empirical data for their ability in explanation and prediction of the multi-faceted phenomena of mental illness and mental health. The definition-decision-making process model would seem to offer a potentially fruitful way of looking at the social network at its point of greatest impact on the person affected.

What this chapter has intended to convey is that community mental health is only a part of the system of services for care; thus workers in that field need to be cognizant of the relationship to all other parts of the system.

Further, one general premise of systems theory offers a potentially large opportunity for workers in the field. That premise suggests that change in any part of the social system will effect change in all other parts. Therefore, the introduction into the community of a mental health center can be expected to affect to some degree all other aspects of that community as a social system. This, too, is a two-sided coin; for example, while improvement may be made in suicide prevention, the question still remains, "What other ramifications will this have for persons and systems in the community?" The question is not idle rhetoric for, as has been shown, the social system of care is all of one piece. To assume independence is to take a short-sighted view and that could mark the community mental movement as nothing more than a fleeting fad in the history of mankind.

What *is* required is a conception of the entire set of systemic relationships and their functional interdependence. Such a view insists that programs be planned and evaluated within such a framework. Failure to use a systems approach is tantamount to professional chauvinism! It is in this spirit that this chapter has been offered. Perhaps it will provide a larger view to community mental health, and, along with that view will come more sensitive and more certain programs and services for the client and for society.

REFERENCES

1. Parsons, T. Structure & Process in Modern Societies. New York, Free Press of Glencoe, 1959.
2. Von Bertalanffy, L.V. General System Theory. New York, Braziller, 1968.
3. Buckley, W. ed. Modern Systems Research for the Behavioral Scientists. Chicago, Aldine Publishing Co., 1968.
4. The General Systems Approach: Contributionf Forward on Holistic Conception of Social Work. Hearn, G., ed. Council on Social Work Education, New York.
5. Lindman, F.T., and McIntyre, D.M., The Mentally Disabled and the Law. Chicago, University of Chicago Press, 1961.
6. Action for Mental Health: Final Report of the Joint Commission on Mental Illness and Health. New York, Basic Books, Inc., 1961.
7. Ibid., p. 136.
8. McCann, The Churches and Mental Health.
9. Schwartz, M., and Schwartz, C.G. Social Approaches to Mental Patient Care, New York, Columbia University Press, 1964, p. 103.
10. Lindeman and McIntyre, op. cit..
11. Mechanic, D. Some factors in identifying and defining mental illness, Ment. Hyg., 46:66-74, January, 1962.
12. Scheff, T. Being Mentally Ill, A Sociological Theory, Chicago, Aldine Publishing Company, 1966, p. 149.
13. Action for Mental Health, op. cit., p. 286.
14. Fuchs, V.R., The contribution of health services to the american economy. Milbank Memorial Fund Quarterly, XLIV, Oct. 1966, p. 85.
15. Goffman, E. Stigma, Notes on the Management of Spoiled Identity. Englewood Cliffs, New Jersey, Prentice-Hall, Inc., 1963.
16. Muth, L.T. Aftercare Services for the Mentally Ill, Mimeographed, 1957. Available from the Mental Health Education Unit, Smith, Kline and French Laboratories, Philadelphia, Pennsylvania.
17. Ibid., p. 63.
18. Health Organizations, Agencies and Schools. Hospitals, 39, Part 2, August 1, 1965.
19. Davis, K. Mental hygiene and the class structure, Psychiatry, 1:55-65. Feb. 1938.
20. Seeley, J. Social values, the mental health movement, and mental health, Ann. Amer. Acad. Political Soc. Sci., 286:15-24, March, 1953.
21. Gursslin, O., Hunt, R., and Roach, J. Social class and the mental health movement. Social Problems, 7, No. 3. pp. 210-218. 1960.
22. Jahoda, M. Current Concepts of Positive Mental Health, New York Basic Books, Inc., 1958, p. 119.
23. Gurin, G., Feld, S., and Veroff, D. Americans View Their Mental Health, New York, Basic Books, Inc., 1957.
24. Cumming, E., and Cumming, J.H. Affective symbolism, social norms and mental illness, Psychiatry, XIX, No. 1, pp. 77-85., 1956.
25. Seeley, J. et al. New York, Basic Books, Inc. 1965, p. 410.

26. Seeley, loc. cit.
27. Cumming, E., and Cumming, J.H. Closed Ranks; An experiment in mental health education, Cambridge, Massachusetts, Harvard University Press, 1957.
27. Goffman, E. Stigma, Notes on the Management of Spoiled Identity, Englewood Cliffs, New Jersey, Prentice-Hall, Inc., 1963.
28. Scheff, op. cit.
29. Scheff, loc. cit., pp. 96-97.
30. Becker, H.S. Outsiders; Studies in the sociology of Deviance, New York, Free Press, 1963.
31. Mills, C.W. The Sociological Imagination. New York, The Grove Press, 1961, pp. 8-9.
32. Goffman, E. Asylums. New York, Doubleday & Company, Inc., 1961, p. 140 ff.
33. Scheff, T. Social conditions for rationality: how urban and rural courts deal with the mentally ill. Amer. Behav. Sci., 7:21-27, March, 1964.
34. Kutner, L. The illusion of due process in commitment proceedings, Northwestern Univ. Law Rev., 57:383-99 September–October, 1962.
35. Wenger, D. A confrontation of professions: the medical-legal debate, and the effect of legal counsel on the commitment decision, Sociologics, 3, No. 1, pp. 23-35. (Published by Alpha Kappa Delta, Department of Sociology, the Ohio State University.)
36. Goffman, E. Asylums. New York, Doubleday-Anchor, 1961, p. 140 ff. See especially footnotes 7, 8, and 9, pp. 131-133.
37. Ibid.
38. Sampson, H., Messinger, S., and Towne, R.D. Family processes and becoming a mental patient. Amer. J. Sociol., 68:88-96. 1962.
39. Sampson, H. Messinger, S., Towne, R.D. and Ross, D., Livson, F., Bowers, M.D., Cohen, L., Dorst, K.S. The mental hospital and marital family ties. Social Problems, IX, Fall, 1961, pp. 141-155.
40. Bredemeier, H.C. The socially handicapped and the agencies. In Reissman, L. et al., eds. Mental Health of the Poor. New York, Free Press of Glencoe, 1964, pp. 88-109.

Social Power in Community Psychiatric Nursing

ANITA WERNER O'TOOLE, R.N., PH.D.

Community psychiatric nursing is based on some type of theory of social power. The phenomenon of power is present in all organizational relationships; in fact, it is never completely absent from any social interaction.[1] Whether a nurse interacts with patients, other nurses, or other professionals, she operates within a context of social power. Her understanding of such theory often is implicit and her use of interventions based on a theory of power is therefore, intuitive. Elaboration of theories of social power have value to the nurse practioner because it helps her to systematically order those factors in her practice that are related to a concept of power. Consequently, intervention becomes more explicit and thus is subject to formulation and subsequent testing of its value. In addition, the use of an explicit analysis of power in practice is useful to refine, expand, and validate a concept. Much of what is called theory in social science is still in the preliminary stages of conceptualization, and often seems to be lost in a fog of analytic debates and disagreements regarding definitional disputes. What is needed is a union of practice and theory in order to improve both.

In this paper I will focus on a general discussion of sociological and social psychological theories of power and show how these may be useful to psychiatric nurses in community settings. The concept of power takes on relevance in community psychiatric nursing when for example, one considers the multitude of problems confronting a profession caught in the midst of a social movement leading to drastic changes in the delivery of mental health care. Realignment of traditional professional roles, reassessment of standard treatment modalities, and development of new organizational formats are just a few of the tasks that face nurses who work in community settings; all of them are intricately involved with issues of power.

Concerns directly related to clients also involve elements of power. Recently, certain client groups have adopted power maneuvers successfully used by other minority groups, in order to get demands met. Examples are the demonstrations of mothers on welfare and the student "sit-ins" in colleges across the country. Both of these client groups are employing bold power tactics which lead to confrontations, and are making it imperative that those who are in a position to negotiate with them understand power. Although mentally ill persons so far have not organized to the extent necessary to confront and change inequities in their care, there is no guarantee that they will not do so. Perhaps what is needed for this relatively powerless group is the intervention of professional workers who can become their advocates by forcing change in communities to allow for more adequate care. Nurses must understand power to participate in this movement.

Since the time of Machiavelli, the question of power has occupied a central position in social theory.[2] Whether or not early social philosophers viewed power as a central dynamic in human relationships depended on their view of the nature of man. When they viewed man as essentially evil, as did Machiavelli and Hobbes then they deemed it necessary to establish order in a chaotic world by instituting power by force.[3-4] However, when they viewed mankind as basically good, as did Rousseau and Moore, they tended to see order as intrinsically inherent in social groupings.[5-6] The problem then was one of maintaining order by other means than force or coercion.

Modern social theorists do not see power in such absolute terms. Even in present day versions of social power, there remains however an implicit assumption that man tends to use power universally in social relationships to control his environment and thus get what he wants or needs. Marwell states this well in a summary of the notions of Blau and Thibaut and Kelly:

> These theorists start with the assumption that all persons seek to so structure their physical and social environment through their behavior that they attain a high potential for getting what they want out of their environment. This potential . . . is here termed social power.[7]

Two basic points are implied in this definition about the concept of power on which there is general agreement among sociologists.[8] The first point is that social power is always the *potential* for action, but not the actual exercise of that potential. Secondly, power is determined by the interrelationship of persons in a social organization; it is not based simply on qualities possessed by the person who holds power. This means that an individual or a group is powerful only in relation to other individuals or groups who have less power. Power thus implies reciprocity between the person in power and those who are submissive to him. An obvious illustration of this point is seen when one considers that a king could not be a king without a kingdom, that is, subjects who recognize his right to be a king.

Even though there is general agreement that power is the potential for action, there is considerable disagreement as to the form of this action. Bierstedt defines power in action as latent force, force as manifest power, and authority as institutionalized power.[9] According to his view, power becomes authority when it is institutionalized in a formal organization by means of the sanctions accorded the power wielders by those who submit to the power. Power becomes force when it is uninstitutionalized and operates in the formal aspect of an organization.

Buckely takes issue with Bierstedt for his failure to maintain analytic distinctions between the concepts of authority and power. He defines these two concepts in the following way:

> *As a suggested working definition, we may define power as control or influence over the actions of others to promote one's goals without their consent, against their 'will,' or without their knowledge or understanding (for example, by control of the physical, psychological, or sociocultural environment within which others must act) . . . .*
>
> *Authority is the direction or control of the behavior of others for the promotion of collective goals, based on some ascertainable form of their knowledgeable consent. . . . As defined, authority is not a special form of power, nor is power a subtype of authority.*[10]

MacIver made this distinction also when he defined authority in terms of the established *right* within a social group of one man to act as a leader to other men.[11] The necessity for this right to be legitimized which leads to a further issue: group consensus or dissensus regarding the predominant goal orientation of the group. When members agree on the group goal or goals, a state of cooperation exists wherein authority to guide the group is seen as legitimate. Conversely, dissensus regarding group goals creates a competitive situation leading to a power structure often based on coercion. Of course, neither of these two extreme conditions exists to the exclusion of the other. Every social group contains elements of both cooperation and competition; however, when one or the other prevails a predominance of either legitimate authority or power also is seen.[12-13]

The mechanisms by which power is exercised to control others against their will may range from brute physical force and manipulation of symbols and information to the dispensing of conditional rewards.[14] Such rewards may be in the form of money, property, prestige, or status. Secord and Backman further suggest that the controlled or influenced person must be dependent on resources or rewards and, furthermore, must have no other alternative source of the desired resources.[15] For example, an employee who is dependent for his survival on his wages is in a potentially powerless position relative to his employer, but only if there are no other available sources of income.

In summarizing the preceding discussion of social power, it is important to keep in mind the conceptual distinction made between power and authority. Often the behavior associated with these two concepts appears the same; acts which direct, control, or influence characterize both power and authority. However, one must look beyond the immediate behavior and examine more closely the motivation or purpose of the controlling act and its ultimate consequences. To define authority merely in terms of institutionalization, as Bierstedt suggests, implies a sanctioning of the norms of an institution by its members, a sanctioning which often does not exist. There may be a fine line of distinction (but an important one), between acquiescense to enforced rules and active consensus regarding organizational norms. Such a distinction is crucial, however, if conceptual clarity is to be achieved and if utilization of these concepts in practice is to be facilitated.

Authority, then, may be distinguished from power when the acts of control are for the purpose of promoting collective goals rather than private or individualistic goals. Furthermore, there must be some evidence that there is explicit awareness or knowledge of these collective goals and the means designed to achieve them. On the other hand, power often depends on concealment or disguise of ultimate goals.

RELEVANCE TO NURSING

In the remainder of this paper I will consider the specific ways that power and authority are relevant to psychiatric nursing in community settings. It is not my purpose to take a moral stand against the use of power. It seems that both power and authority have their relative merits when used appropriately and with a high degree of awareness. It *is* my purpose, however, to aid in the acquisition of this heightened awareness among nurses who may find themselves in the position to choose between power and authority.

Working with people who are mentally ill has always involved elements of power. In part, this is so because often people who suffer from mental illness also suffer from a sense of powerlessness and hopelessness. This attitude gets transferred to the staff who, in order to ward off feelings of powerlessness in themselves, may respond with distorted notions about their own ability to transform or influence patients. Textbooks on traditional psychotherapies repeatedly emphasize the importance for the therapist to avoid an omnipotent attitude toward patients.

Power maneuvers among staff serve to render the patient more powerless than he was initially. A reciprocal interactive response is set into motion wherein one group tries to outdo another in power maneuvers. Patients, as well as staff, can be controlling in this struggle. The patient who is incontinent, physically abusive, provocative, or simply uncooperative holds a manipulative type of power over staff that is often unexcelled by other types of power relationships.

Another factor that involves psychiatric workers in issues of power is the patient's lack of awareness, at times, that he has a problem. Then the therapist must assume a position of control or influence against the will of the patient. This position has always been rationalized by reassurances that the professional worker knows best what will help the patient and, in due time, the patient will "see the light" and appreciate the care given him. Sometimes this has been the case, but at other times the patient leaves the hospital with his problem untouched and without acceptance of the idea that the "medicine was good for him."

In the last few years there has been some attempt in psychiatry to change some of the hierarchical patterns of organizing care to diminish the problems of unequal power positions between staff members and patients. The first such movement was embodied in the therapeutic milieu philosophy where existing organizational systems of psychiatric care were changed to approximate more closely a democratic system with its attendant flattening of hierarchical role structures. This democratization of organizational systems tended to open new avenues for nurses to participate more as equal team members; thus, in some instances, the nurse was free to move into a system of cooperative team endeavor. However, such movements often created new problems by disguising issues of power under ideological tenets of equality that were only spoken and not acted upon.

Movement into the community was a logical outgrowth of the therapeutic milieu movement. Both were based on the assumption that mental illness is social in etiology and thus could be treated most effectively by manipulating the social conditions of the patient. In a community setting, the nurse has the opportunity to influence more aspects of the patient's life than she had in most therapeutic milieu programs. To the extent that such intervention is accepted by the patient, the nurse is accorded considerable authority to influence the patient's life. At the same time, the nurse working in the community has less control over the environment she works in. She makes home visits, contacts clients in public places, visits schools, and so on. In such settings she has far less control over the environment than she did in the hospital. Whether or not this situation leads to the development of new power tactics to insure the comfort of the nurse will depend on the degree of interpersonal competence she has acquired.

The power position of the patient—or potential patient—also changes in the community setting. Patients can refuse to come to agencies for services or, once there they can refuse to accept the services offered. Few agencies can survive without the important resource of a clientele, and one way to avoid this problem is to engage in case-finding. Instead of the person coming to the agency for assistance, the staff go out and look for people who need help.

Although this practice represents an effort to fulfill the mandate of community psychiatry—to promote mental health and prevent mental illness—it also raises new problems. It increases the power of psychiatry to define persons as mentally ill. According to Leifer:

> A substantial degree of the psychiatrist's power is based on his ability to socially deface an individual by 'diagnosing' him as 'mentally ill' and, in effect, to imprison him by means of psychiatric commitment. The modification of psychiatric hospitals under the community psychiatry mandate does not alter their function [16]

This raises the question of the basis for definition of mental illness. As psychiatry moves more and more into the arena of social control by defining deviant behavior as illness, there must be a concomitant and clear recognition of the social power involved in that endeavor.

Nurses working in the community have increased opportunities to work directly with patients, and to participate in diagnosis and therapy utilizing a variety of treatment modalities. In order to assume this increased responsibility, nurses must be aware of the increased authority and power which accompanies it, and must be prepared to assume the responsibility with rational judgement based on knowledge and competence.

REFERENCES

1. Bierstedt, R., An analysis of social power. Amer. Socio. Rev., 15:730-738, 1950.
2. Machiavelli, N. The Prince. Intro. by Caponigri, A.R., Chicago, Regnery, 1963.
3. Ibid.
4. Hobbes, T. Leviathan. Randall, F.B., ed. New York, Washington Square Press, 1958.
5. Rousseau, J. Social Contract. New York, E.P. Dutton Co., 1950.
6. Moore, T. Utopia. Collins, J.C., ed. Oxford, Oxford University Press, 1904.
7. Marwell, G. Adolescent powerlessness and delinquent behavior. Social Prob., 14:35-47, 1966.
8. Smith, T.E. Foundations of parental influence upon adolescents: an application of social power theory. Amer. Socio. Rev., 35:860-873, 1970.
9. Bierstedt, R., op. cit.
10. Buckley, W. Sociology and Modern Systems Theory. Englewood Cliffs, N.J., Prentice-Hall, Inc., 1967, p. 186.
11. MacIver, R. The Web of Government. New York, The MacMillan Company, 1947.
12. Blau, P.M. Cooperation and competition in a bureaucracy. Amer. J. Sociol., 59:6,(May) 530-535, 1954.
13. Gouldner, A. Patterns of Industrial Bureaucracy. New York, Free Press of Glencoe, Inc., 1954.

14. Buckley, op. cit., p. 186.
15. Secord, P.F., and Backman, C.W. Social Psychology. New York, McGraw-Hill Book Company, 1964.
16. Leifer, R. Community Psychiatry and Social Power. Social Problems, 14:17:22, 1966.
17. Thibaut, J.W., and Kelley, H.H. The Social Psychology of Groups. New York, John Wiley & Sons, Inc., 1959.

Stability and Change in Community Mental Health Practice

EUGENE B. NADLER, Ph. D.

The community mental health movement today is a crucible in which previously held thought about mental health is subjected to a searing and purifying heat. On one side, the heat results from the uneasy but salutory collaboration of different mental health professions, and from the quality and magnitude of the tasks the movement has set for itself. On the other side, purification produces theoretical reorientations, with certain psychological ideas being seen as totally inadequate, others as seriously limited and limiting, still others as useful only when connected with other ideas. Theoretical stock taking has been going on for some time[1, 3] the proposed theory must pass muster in at least the following respects:

1. It must be a theory of the normal as well as the abnormal.
2. It must be a theory of psychological stability as well as psychological change.
3. It must be an individual as well as a social theory.
4. It must be a theory of prevention as well as therapy.

The theory that I propose is called "attitude theory," because it owes its greatest debt to the experimental study of attitude functioning that has gone on for over 30 years. It also owes a great deal to the formulations of Boulding,[5] Chein,[7] Kelly,[16] Leeper and Madison,[18] Phillips,[25] and Secord and Backman.[29] Finally, the theory has been shaped by much in the current Zeitgeist as well as by my own clinical experience, which spans both individual and social problems.

ATTITUDE THEORY

Let us start with behavior, with man as an actor in the real world. Nothing, apparently, could be simpler. But behavior is not a simple idea, as examination of even the simplest act will show.

A man goes downtown to buy theater tickets. What is he doing? He is going downtown to buy theater tickets. This characterization of his behavior is in terms of his *intended purpose*. He is foregoing his usual reading of the evening paper. This characterization of his behavior is in terms of an ordered set of personal priorities, a subjective *hierarchy of purposes*. He is becoming the kind of person who invests time, energy, and money in the theater, as opposed to, perhaps, financial speculation. This characterization is in terms of his *potential change of identity*. He is going into an area of high smog and is further befouling his already befouled lungs. This characterization is in terms of its *unwanted and unintended consequences*. He is gratifying the wishes of theater people. This characterization of his behavior is in terms of its *immediate social consequences*. He is putting money into circulation, thus changing the economic environment in which he lives. This characterization is in terms of its *ultimate social consequences*. He is creating the potential for conflict with his working-class neighbors, who don't share the values of the theater, and the potential for relations of harmony with middle-class individuals who are not presently his neighbors. This characterization is in terms of its *potential social consequences*.

I could go on and on. The point is, however, that behavior is not merely a set of muscle twitches. It contains elements both intended and unintended, both in the selfsame act. It includes the purposes of the individual as well as objects outside him. It is fractionated and organized in nested hierarchies of itself. Originating in the individual, it inevitably has social meaning and consequences.

Confronted by the staggering complexity of behavior, we try to make a beginning by separating out the main elements, slowing down the action, and reconstructing, in imagination, a schematic form.

Imagine that the mind of a person is a computer and inside that computer is a set of programs. The programs process incoming information and send out behavior. The computer thus has both a perceptual and a motor end. The important part of the "computer," however, is the part that contains the programs.

In any given cycle a computer is critically dependent for what it "sees" on the programs that are activated by incoming information. Since the computer cannot do anything for which it is not programmed, it is at the same time critically dependent on the programs for what it does—but not completely.

Although perhaps it is less obvious, the incoming information that activates these computer programs is equally important. This information determines which of the many available programs get activated. If the behavior of the computer can be altered by changing its programs, it also can be altered by changing the information that is fed to it.

THE HUMAN COMPUTER

Again making an analogy to the mind of man, the programs of the computer become beliefs, concepts, plans, interests, loyalties, motives, and attitudes. It may be objected that computers and men are very different things, and computer programs do not work like the mental programs of men. However, the mind-computer does not work like present day computers. It works like a man. The precise problem is to understand the human computer.

Reactivity is the mode of existence of present-day mechanical computers; activity is the mode of existence of the human computer. I do not mean to imply that the human computer does not react to changes in the environment, but that such reactions occur in the context of ongoing behavior. This is related to a second important difference between human and present day mechanical computers, a difference first noted by Chein;[7] the "plans" of present-day mechanical computers are the fixed end-product of the activation of pre-determined programs; human computers must change their programs in order to realize their plans. They change themselves at every moment as a condition of their existence.

One further note to extend the usefulness of the computer model. The human computer exists in a society of other computers, as well as in an inanimate environment which also may be thought of as a computer with particular programming. Its perceptual end is hooked up to the motor end of other computers—to sets, subsets, and individuals. By the same token, the motor end of the human computer is hooked up to perceptual end of other computers. In this way the computers influence each other by activating each others' programs. The whirring of computers and their mutual influence is a first approximation to the behavior of man in the real world.

Hypothesis 1

A person's mind is filled with latent behaviors, among which are those formations we call attitudes.

The hypothesis of mind is not one I will spend much time proving. I concur with Singer that mind is behavior that will occur in the future.[30] The hypothesis of mind seems to be required by the behavior of people, but not by the behavior of rocks. This proof will be convincing to all but the most thoroughgoing behaviorists.

I include attitudes among the contents of the mind because large portions of the social behavior of men are social from the very first activation of latent behaviors. These mental programs take other people into account from the moment that they become active; they are oriented toward other people and refer to them. An attitude is an implicit statement, an ideal if you will, of the kind of relationship a person wishes to have with some aspect of his social surroundings. It is aimed directly and explicitly at other people or at social objects. Most of the behavior of fathers, bosses, buyers, representatives, and teachers is guided by such attitudes, and cannot be reduced to other behaviors.

Characterizing these mental elements as "wished-for social relationships" defines attitudes at a high level of abstraction. However it does cover the spectrum—from the social motives involved in two-person interaction through those, for example, of a corporation president handling his company—to the worship of deities. It avoids the reductionist error, yet is less schematic than concepts proposed by other mental health workers—the "assertion" of Phillips,[25] the "personal construct" of Kelly,[16] the "personality habit" of Leeper and Madison,[18] the "images" of Boulding[5] and Tomkins.[32] The "attitude" of the social psychologist connotes something more emotional than an assertion, more purposive than a habit, more social than a construct, and more long-range than the personality theorist's favorite, the motive. It also implies an object, situation, or set of objects and situations in the real world. This reminds us that however much men may introspect and ruminate, their main psychological activity is oriented toward dealing with the real world.

The inclusion of specifically social contents among the elements of mind is required not only by a social psychology, but also by an abnormal psychology. What has been learned of neurosis and psychosis shows that social attitudes are usually (perhaps always) heavily implicated, which is not the same as saying that they are *the* cause. We have in mind such attitudes as grandiosity, submissiveness, fear of intimacy, sexual inhibitions, authoritarianism, suspiciousness, alienation, and so on. These are implicated in individual pathology, just as attitudes of racial and religious prejudice, class snobbery, bureaucracy, and political manipulativeness and coerciveness are implicated in social pathology. Recent work on social factors in mental illness[12, 20, 31] shows some of the empirical connections between individual and social pathology, connections our theory must take into account.

Hypothesis 2

There is room in the mind for additional latent behaviors, including attitudes.

The evidence that people learn is impressive. Older children know more and do more than younger children, and adults know and do more than either. The evidence seems to be that people continue to learn throughout life. Furthermore, it is possible to learn in all areas of life, from the formal learning that goes on in settings requiring novel forms of socialization, to the creative learning that goes on in artistic and scientific settings. Without specifying the mechanism of this learning, our second hypothesis makes explicit the possibility.

Hypothesis 3

The latent behaviors of the mind are hierarchically organized, such that a quantitative value can be assigned to each element.

There are at least two reasons for believing that the mind is hierarchically organized, and that in some subjective sense certain elements are more important than others. One is that people seem to spend more time and energy in certain pursuits than in others. On a mass scale, the problem of sheer biological survival occupies a predominant place in the thought and action of most people in the underdeveloped world. That is not true of people in the advanced countries, where other interests loom larger. At the individual level, we see that some people are preoccupied with money, others with friendship, still others with the satisfactions of a craft. Even granting that, to some degree, priorities arise out of situations, the patterning of choices in relatively free-choice situations indicates that some priorities are internal.

The second reason is that people can and do make decisions where decisions require a choice between conflicting alternatives. The case where people stand suspended between apparently equal alternatives is exceptional and provides an occasion for literary speculation or psychiatric intervention. By and large, the decisions that people make are made relatively easily, although not necessarily correctly. I suggest that the reason for this derives from the hierarchical organization of the mind, in which conflicting alternatives are rarely equal.

Hypothesis 4

When a behavior is active, the person tends to seek confirmation of that behavior.

This is the most important hypothesis of attitude theory. It was first stated by Phillips in what must be considered a sadly neglected book.[25] If we generalize the concepts of confirmation and disconfirmation to include not only the phenomena of abnormal psychology, but also the phenomena of social attitudes and social process, we develop an extremely powerful concept.

Confirmation is a generic term meaning goal attainment in the case of such items as attitudes, interests, plans, loyalties, and motives; verification in the case of such items as beliefs, opinions, and concepts, and changing the situation in preconceived ways in all cases. In the strict sense, confirmation means engaging in behavior that supports, serves, and is included in other behavior.

One way in which the tendency toward confirmation shows itself is in the behavior of people in ambiguous situations. Even when clear guidelines are lacking, people still behave in goal-directed (although not necessarily appropriate), ways. Under such conditions, the selectivity of thought and perception are seen quite clearly. I suggest that this selectivity is an expression of the tendency to seek to confirm whatever latent behaviors have been aroused.

Other expressions of the tendency to seek confirmation are: (1) the tendency to remember that which serves one's present purposes; (2) the tendency to seek out people whose views are similar to one's own; and (3) the tendency to read books in line with one's own interests and values. Many of the phenomena of abnormal psychology may also be seen in this way—delusions and hallucinations which serve a particular attitude, "defenses" which are erected to protect a particular view of the world, the tendency to manipulate people in ways that will confirm the opinions and attitudes that are held concerning them.

Hypothesis 4A

Pleasant emotions result from confirmation of behavior, unpleasant emotions from disconfirmation.

This hypothesis sees emotion mainly as a by-product of behavior, a phenotype. Some apparently peculiar facts make sense when viewed in its light.

Why do radically prejudiced individuals often have very positive feelings for certain members of the group they "dislike?" Hypothesis 4A suggests that it is because these members behave in such a way as to confirm a wished-for social relationship—they are the "good Negroes," the "white Jews," and so on, the ones who "know their place." Attitudes are concerned with place; emotions derive from keeping or not keeping place.

Why do depressed individuals exude such a peculiar joy in being miserable? We suggest that their self-punishing behavior confirms a poor self-image. Phillips has suggested that the preponderantly pleasant memories that most people have would be inverted in the case of depressed individuals if confirmation rather than the pleasure principle were operating.[25]

Why do apparently pleasant feelings like sex and joy disturb some individuals? Because such feelings are inconsistent with a set of attitudes roughly described as "puritan." The pleasure principle, however, would make precisely the opposite prediction.

Once emotions are generated, of course, they do become "causes" of behavior, as positive and negative feedback mechanisms[19]. But this is secondary from a conceptual standpoint.

Hypothesis 5

The quantitative value, the place in the mental hierarchy, of a latent behavior is a function of the amount of confirmation it has received.

The idea presented in this hypothesis superficially resembles the behavioristic idea of reinforcement. For example, if I believe the earth is round, and my friends believe it, if authorities on the subject believe it, and if all written statements I've encountered subscribe to it, then the chances are I will hold this belief pretty firmly; in other words, it will occupy a position high on my mental hierarchy. The resemblance of Hypothesis 5 to the idea of reinforcement is only superficial, however.

Confirmation means engaging in behavior that serves other behavior, the latter being instrumental to the former. What is confirmed is an end, and the behavior that confirms it is a means. The more I invest in the idea of the earth being round, the more important a place it occupies in my mental hierarchy. In fact, the idea is very similar to the psychoanalytic idea of investment. If there is any law of effect operating, it would have to be called an inverse law of effect.

The strongest direct evidence for this hypothesis comes from experiments which show that the more effort it takes to learn a behavior, the stronger and more resistant to change is that behavior[9, 18]. It is also possible to interpret most of the research on partial reinforcement in this way. Finally, there are the experiments of Festinger and his followers which show that trapping people into supporting positions contrary to their values produces more value change than directly convincing them for good substantial reasons.[10, 17] Presumably, much more effort goes into the former.

In addition, there is the speculative grist provided by the "boomerang effect" which has been observed in experiments on attitude change. Propaganda or counterarguments designed to change certain attitudes often have the opposite effect of strengthening them. The theory of reinforcement cannot be operating, since a counterargument can at best be interpreted as a non-reinforcement, at worst a punishment. Hypothesis 5, as well as some empirical investigation, reveals that arguments boomerang when the person is somehow able to alter their impact so that they confirm his attitudes. We may extend this reasoning to psychotherapeutic interpretations that do not "take;" the person has transformed their meaning, and thus strengthened his dysfunctional behavior.

Hypothesis 5 tells us that not only are people behaving and making decisions all the time—on the basis of a set of mental priorities—but the basis of these decisions is constantly altered with every decision made.

Hypothesis 6

When behaviors which confirm each other are active, they form a new unit whose value in the hierarchy is some function of the sum of their separate values.

The evidence for this hypothesis comes mostly from the studies of the Gestalt psychologists. Heider, particularly, has made use of the idea of unit formation: "Separate entities comprise a unit when they are perceived as belonging together," (11, p. 176) What Heider has omitted is a conception of the quantitative power of such a unit in the behavioral, actually the decision-making, process.

The dethroning of Stalin in the minds of the Russian people provides a nice example of summation effects in unit formation. Stalin had achieved such stature in the minds of the Russians that his image remained upshaken during the whole long period when it was being disconfirmed by rumors and by Western propaganda. When Khruschev came along and added his prestige to these rumors and propaganda, the psychological weight shifted. The conflict for the Russians and for the world communists could only be resolved by downgrading Stalin. This brings us to our next hypothesis.

Hypothesis 7

When behaviors which disconfirm each other are active those of lesser value are reorganized in the service of those of higher value.

A piece of information can be used to change an attitude only if it somehow occupies a higher place in the mental hierarchy of the target person. Prestige suggestion will work only if the prestige person has enough prestige in the mind of the target person, or if he can add to his weight by aligning himself with important elements. The timing of a therapeutic interpretation is important because it must come at a moment when the person has already amassed independent evidence of its correctness.

The "boomerang effects" we spoke of awhile ago are not exceptions to Hypothesis 7; they conform to it. The experimenter or therapist who lofts a counterargument against one of a person's attitudes may think it quite powerful—the attitude must surely give way. But if it is less powerful than the attitude, then the counterargument will be altered to serve the attitude. The important question is the position the counterargument will occupy in the mind of the target person in relation to that of the attitude in question.

It is this question of hierarchical position that is omitted from most of the balance and dissonance theories of attitude change. (The theories of Osgood and Tannenbaum are an exception.)[24] These theories (balance and dissonance) state that when two ideas are in conflict, one or the other must give way to reduce the dissonance. By assigning quantitative values to these ideas, we can predict, at least in principle, not only that attitude change will occur, but also the direction of change.

Further, the process of change is actually identical with the process of behaving. Here we acknowledge our debt to Chein who has pointed out that a motive is a behavior that subsumes other behaviors.[7] In order to type I must sit; I cannot stand. Sitting is thus included in typing, serves typing, and is subordinate to typing. To achieve the purpose of typing, I must change my behavior from standing to sitting. The conflict between standing and typing is resolved in favor of sitting and typing. Stability and change are thus inherent in the simplest acts; to stabilize typing I must alter my position.

Hypothesis 7 is also an extention of Hypothesis 4 which speaks of the tendency toward confirmation. The process of behaving always involves conflict between opposing behaviors each seeking confirmation. When one changes in the interests of the other, the latter is thereby confirmed. Thus behavior change itself is an expression of the tendency toward confirmation. The statement of these as separate principles is for purposes of clarity of exposition.

Hypothesis 7A

When behaviors which are disconfirmed by the sheer absence of instrumental latent behaviors are active, there will be attempts to develop and learn these latent behaviors.

I have pointed out elsewhere that disconfirmation seems to trigger the mechanism of physiological arousal, or what Pavlov long ago termed the "orienting" or "what-is-it" reflex.[23, 26] The experiments of Jacobson show increasing sensory sensitivity and what might be called "cognitive scanning."[15] Unpleasant emotions increase, and there is increased physiological readiness for action. Other experiments with animals show increases in exploratory and manipulative reactions.[26]

These changes powerfully favor learning, the development of new behavior, or change in behavior. In fact, it has been suggested that Hull's D is the same as generalized arousal.[21] Increasing sensitivity means that the person is more likely to notice environmental changes. Increases in conscious, imaginative, and reflective activity mean that the person makes available to himself more ideas and concepts that may be transferred or brought to bear on the problem. The increasing readiness for action and the enlargement of the scope of exploratory behavior means that the person is more likely to try something new, to experiment, to change his environment so that he receives even more new information from it. And the emotions that are aroused are motivating; they keep the person at it. Other behaviors superordinate to the behavior that has been disconfirmed may be thereby aroused, resulting in the change of that behavior.

Learning and development is thus seen as a special case of intrapsychic conflict resolution. We may take as a model the following example. The learner is embarked on some enterprise, that is, he is behaving with a goal in mind. He may be trying to hold onto a job, create a political organization, pursue some moral imperative. He finds himself blocked by his own ignorance, that is, by behaviors with respect to particular objects that are incomplete, inappropriate, or so badly organized that they impede the attainment of his goals. If he changes certain behaviors, generates new ones, and reorganizes others in order to attain his goals, then he has learned. The novel behaviors take their place in the unused part of his mind. Or, during the process of arousal, the person may discover higher purposes that dictate changes in the behavior that got him started in the first place. In both cases, whether the goal is old or new, learning, development and change confirm the goal and the conflict is resolved, since the conflict between the goal and the means to its attainment has been erased. At one and the same time, this resolution of "intrapsychic" conflict in turn resolves a conflict between a person and his environment.

The theory I have outlined views every act as expressive of a conflict between superordinate and subordinate behaviors. In every act, there is confirmation of some behavior and change in other behavior. In every act pleasant and unpleasant emotions are generated—pleasant feelings from the behavior that is confirmed, unpleasant ones from the behavior that is disconfirmed. Every act is also a decision, a choice between competing behaviors, thus influencing the outcome of future decisions. And finally, every act contains elements of both tradition and novelty in which we both realize ourselves and create ourselves.

SOME DERIVATIONS REGARDING MENTAL DISORDER

We begin by noting that, by and large, people tend to develop attitudes that are appropriate to the situations they are in. Indeed, this seems to be the meaning of the different outlooks of people of different nationality, religion, social class, milieu, and so on. We might almost say, as an ideal statement, that if a person is in a given situation long enough, he will eventually develop attitudes that stand a high chance of being confirmed in that situation, in other words, that are realistic.

As we have seen, this is a far from passive process. In making these adaptations, each individual brings to his problem attitudes developed in previous situations that are similar. In applying these attitudes, he experiences some disconfirmation. To some extent these attitudinal residues are altered to suit the new situation; to some extent the new situation is bent to suit the old residues. These attitudinal residues are themselves residues of previous adaptations, so that the adaptation and the attitude that the person achieves in a given situation represent a large portion of his previous psychological history, refracted through the lens of his present situation. It is these attitudinal residues, these latent behaviors formed in previous contexts, each seeking confirmation, that makes adaptation an active rather than a passive process.

The trouble is that situations just do not remain stationary, especially in the modern world. Psychoanalytic work has established the inappropriateness to the adult situation of many attitudes developed in childhood. The anthropologist Benedict has made the same point for many social macrocosms in her discussion of cultural discontinuity.[4] We must extend this thinking to include such generalizations as the following: the attitudes developed on one job may be inappropriate to the next; different attitudes may be required as one changes one's status with respect to age, marital status, region or residence, social and economic condition, and the timeless vicissitudes of life—accident, disease, and death. The world constantly disconfirms our attitudes about it; new attitudes and new adaptations are always necessary.

Derivation 1

A person's potential for mental disorder consists of the presence in his mind of relatively important attitudes which stand little change of being confirmed.

At the root of mental disorder we find, not something *in* the person, but a relationship between the person and his environment. On the one hand there is an attitude seeking confirmation; on the other is a refractory environment. An adult person who is as dependent as a child is unlikely to confirm his dependency in his relationships with other people. A person at the bottom levels of society is unlikely to find even ordinary respect accorded him among status-oriented, class-conscious people.

In order for an attitude to exhibit potentiality for mental disorder, however, it must be high on the person's hierarchy of latent behaviors. The food preferences of most people are far down the ladder of their mental hierarchies. This is not true of Orthodox Jews or religious Hindus; difficulties in satisfying the food preferences of the latter could produce real anguish. It is likely that attitudes concerning security, autonomy, sexual identity, and group membership rank quite high with most people.

The mental health worker must have a conception, not only of types of attitudes exhibited by individuals, but of the range of environments these individuals might be exposed to. Every attitude is "appropriate" for some environment. A grandiose, power-oriented person, for example, can confirm his attitudes if he occupies a position of power. But how will he function if he is suddenly shifted to an environment in which he occupies a menial and impotent position? A prognosis concerning the potential for mental disorder must consider the person's attitudes, the rank of these attitudes, and the probability of his being exposed to disconfirming environments. One type of preventive psychiatry for the individual may focus simply on preventing major disconfirmations from occurring.

A more important and basic method of preventive psychiatry attempts to develop a large repertoire of realistic attitudes in relation to anticipated situations that have varying probabilities of occurrence. Here we are close to the "competence" definitions of mental health of Argyris[2] and White.[33] This kind of competence was, historically, precisely what was aimed at in a "liberal education." This was a liberating education that built into the person an array of attitudes so numerous, wide-ranging and complex that it was unlikely that he would encounter too many situations that he could not master. In past times the culture-shock of a trip abroad was widely utilized as a mind-stretcher, as was the religious retreat, the intense struggle of the Socratic dialogue, and the requirement of many progressive schools that high-born young people seek jobs, for a period, in manual occupations and social service. More recently, "far-out" educational forms that are sometimes extremely sophisticated psychologically have made their appearance—sensitivity training, encounters, soul sessions, Zen discipline, happenings, programmed disinhibition, and drug-induced consciousness expansion. Without commenting on the merits of these forms, I will note their common aim of education and reeducation for anticipated situations.

Derivation 2

Symptoms of mental disorder appear when attitudes that are relatively high on a person's hierarchy of latent behaviors are disconfirmed.

Some of the symptoms of mental disorder may be seen in even minor instances of disconfirmation involving relatively unimportant behaviors. I go into my bedroom at night, turning up the light switch as I enter. The light bulb, however, has burned out. I become annoyed, and flick the light switch two or three more times, but the light still does not go on. I finally go for a new bulb.

Here is demonstrated, in low-powered form: (a) the operation of a hopelessly unrealistic expectation; (b) a denial of reality; (c) the repetition compulsion; and (d) the resolution of a conflict by giving up a fixation. If we substitute an unrealistic interpersonal or social attitude for this expectation, and move it up the hierarchy of importance so that it is near the top, we get some idea of the magnitude and quality of a serious mental disorder.

In a recent study I conducted, the hypothesis was tested that disconfirming events are a necessary condition for the development of mental disorder. A group of day hospital patients, mostly psychotic, was compared to a group of normal controls matched for age, sex, social class, and religion. This demographic matching resulted in a personality matching; there was only one significant difference between the two groups on thirty ratings of personality dimensions. This difference accounted for none of the variance of a measure of mental health status. Yet, a measure of recent stresses that could be considered disconfirming on a priori grounds—accident, disease, death in the family, and so on, correlated .71 with criterion of severity of mental illness. When personality is held constant, mental illness becomes almost synonymous with the piling up of disconfirmations in a comparatively short time period.

Regardless of the attitude that underlies the disturbance, so-called "symptoms" seem to fall into three categories. First, there are the phenomena associated with the state of arousal that is triggered by disconfirmation—sensory hypersensitivity, introspection, random and novel behavior, and physiological mobilization. Second, we have the sense of threat to the self arising from the disconfirmation of an important attitude and the unpleasant emotions generated by that. Third, there is the obvious presence of defenses, behavior changes that have occurred in the service of an attitude of paramount importance that maintain that attitude in the face of further disconfirming experience. And finally, there is the persistence of the attitude, its rigidity in the face of disconfirmation, indeed, its strengthening over time as it escalates up the mental hierarchy as more and more experiences are assimilated to it.

In terms of this theory, how might we understand the rough distinction between neurosis and psychosis? We have seen that maintaining an unrealistic attitude involves changing subordinate behaviors in its service, and, as a result, moving the unrealistic attitude up the mental hierarchy. If this process is continued long enough, we cross a threshold where the imperious attitude begins to dissolve extremely basic latent behaviors in its maw—those having to do with perceptual and motor functioning, or what have been called "ego functions." The crossover from neurosis to psychosis is similar to the development of what the old timers used to call a "monomania," a singleminded interest whose stability and growth requires that the person take himself apart psychologically.

Derivation 3

Symptoms of mental disorder disappear under either of two circumstances: (1) when latent behavior that has been disconfirmed is finally confirmed; or (2) when latent behavior that has been disconfirmed is changed so that the new behavior is confirmed.

It ought to go without saying that all kinds of activities of the person can produce a reduction or disappearance of symptoms, in or out of psychotherapy. Derivation 3 suggests two mechanisms within the framework of attitude theory by which this can occur.

The first is perhaps best described metaphorically by the folk-saying "The night is darkest just before the dawn." Here, the attitude that is implicated in the anxious night does not change, but events or the actions of the person himself bring about a confirming dawn; the ship comes in, the boy gets the girl, the far-out idea works, the enemy makes his fatal mistake.

The second mechanism of symptom removal depends on change in the attitude itself. As a man who hated his wife told me as we worked on the problem of his marital relationship, "It looks like I have to start seeing a sick animal as a healthy human being." The removal of symptoms by this mechanism requires the presence or the development of attitudes superordinate to the one in question that can affect a change in the latter.

Let us examine a case furnished by Wolpe[34] and try to understand it from the standpoint of attitude theory:

An attractive woman of 28 was very upset by her lover's growing coolness toward her. This was a pattern she had repeated many times.

Once she gained a man's interest, she would adopt an attitude of extreme dependence and submissiveness. He would find this harder and harder to live with and would finally reject her completely. Wolpe told her how to behave with firmness and to take independent courses of action. She was shown how to counter-attack her nagging mother, and how to deal with her boss and other difficult people. The break in the case came after the ninth interview in which she refused, without explanation or discussion, to make her love a ten pound loan. Soon after she was able to achieve a dignified end of the relationship. Later, with another man, she made a supreme effort to be firm and to be guided only by her own desires, but was unable to carry it through, and allowed herself to be seduced, clearly motivated by her old fear of not pleasing. With further treatment, she was able to resist this man, and found to her surprise that his respect for her increased. She was able to go out with still another man and resist seduction. She was less upset by her mother's nagging, and found that in fact it was diminishing as a result of her greater assertiveness. However, she was starting to be bothered by spending so many evenings at home. After a six week vacation, during which she utilized many opportunities to practice her new-found assertiveness, she began to feel increasingly constructive and less anxious in interpersonal situations. She felt more poised and began to achieve social success for the first time in her life. She was no longer bothered by not going out a lot. While on vacation she met a man she was attracted to, but now her feelings had an independent, adult character. She married him three months later, and two-and-a-half years later was reported to be a happily married mother. (Slightly paraphrased from 34, pp. 127-128.)

What motivations may we realistically attribute to this submissive woman? Undoubtedly she wished to escape from the real shame and rage at herself which her submissive behavior aroused. Probably she wished to be better able to cope with those people who brought these feelings out. Maybe she wanted to please her therapist. Maybe she wanted to get married. The change in her submissive attitude can only be understood in terms of the purposes served by this change. An understanding of these purposes allows us not only to understand why the change took place, but also the content and direction of the change. Plainly, this attitude change (and development) was *instrumental to* and *in the service of* the purposes we have mentioned. Not only is all behavior motivated, according to the widely accepted formula, but so too is all psychological change.

This example also brings out the character of attitude change as a complex decision process. A number of motives and attitudes are at play here, producing relations of harmony in some subsets, and relations of conflict in others. My conjectures about the woman's motives reveal unit-formation between (a) her shame and rage at herself, (b) her wish to cope with difficult people, (c) her wish to get married, and (d) her wish to please her therapist. These motives are all consistent with each other, confirm each other, and augment each other to produce a powerful desire for independence. Standing opposed to these motives were others that also formed a unit—her submissiveness to her mother, her boss, her lovers, as well as her own lack of knowledge about *how* to be assertive. The break in the case came when the motives favoring independence outweighed those favoring submission, producing a different decision in a particular situation than previously. This produced a more differentiated independence motive, and also increased the hierarchical importance of the motives favoring independence, so that further decisions in situations involving questions of independence became easier and easier to make in the right direction.

Attitude theory would suggest that the therapist must determine which particular attitudes of the patient are characteristically disconfirmed in particular situations. He must determine the present and potential line-up latent behaviors favoring change and opposing it, including attitudes toward himself in this calculation. And he must see his role as that of midwife of psychological changes that are already under way in the patient as a result of disconfirming experience.

Summary

There is no mental health problem apart from the problems of the person in his environment. On the one hand there are the person's attitudes by which he comes to grips with his environment; on the other hand there are the environmental possibilities for realizing the purposes embodied in these attitudes. Preventive psychiatry for the individual involves preventing stressful disconfirmation or pre-programming him to deal with likely situations. Therepy for the individual involves helping people to realize healthy attitudes and to change unhealthy ones. The phenomena of mental disorder are continuous with the phenomena of disconfirmation in the day-to-day struggle for adaptation.

SOCIAL PROCESS AND PATHOLOGY

It is possible to look at the interactions that occur between people in terms of confirmation and disconfirmation. For example, to agree with another's expression of his attitude is an act that confirms that attitude. To disagree is to disconfirm it. We have all experienced the increase in pleasant feelings and the lessening of tension that results when others agree with us. We have all experienced the rising unpleasantness, increased tension and perception of a "problem" when others disagree with us. Particular agreements and disagreements, of course have their own special features and circumstances. However, many of their common features stem from the psychological consequences of confirmation and disconfirmation.

In the first stage of an argument, for example, the disconfirmation that each person experiences increases his sensitivity to further disconfirmations, so that elements of the speech, manner, and ideas of the other stand out with greater clarity. Problem-directed thinking begins, guided by the need for confirm one's own attitude and making use of the new elements which have entered the picture. Exploratory behavior also begins, similarly guided by the need to confirm the original attitude. The emotions and tensions that are generated sustain the quest for confirmation, making it difficult to let go of the problem. The impact of disconfirmation in an argument is to widen, through generalized activation, the psychological arena in which the struggle is taking place, and to escalate the attitudes at issue up the mental hierarchies of the participants. If a common superordinate goal cannot be found which can subsume attitude change, then the argument escalates further.

With a widening area of disagreement, more of the attitudes of the participants are placed in jeopardy. The "attitude surface" exposed to potential disconfirmation is enlarged, and a point may be reached where a sense of personal threat develops. This point may be reached earlier if threat words are used in the counterarguments, but basically it is the very cleverness of the counterarguments that produces threat. Rebuttal becomes more and more difficult. The two people no longer hear each other as psychological narrowing occurs. They begin to perceive each other as underhanded, insincere, and perhaps as malevolent and inhuman. When an argument reaches this point, it is no longer attitudes that are at stake, but souls.

Derivation 1

When people come together with different attitudes on issues of common concern, their individual efforts to achieve confirmation result in the production of a social struggle to achieve attitude similiarity or complementarity.

This formulation does not say anything about the form of this social struggle. It may be overt or covert. It may be carried on according to rules of reasonable discourse, or it may be carried on argumentatively, politically, or even violently. Attitudinal concensus is not always arrived at in peaceful or democratic ways.

Derivation 1 covers quite a bit of ground. The struggle it speaks of is characteristic of the process of strangers getting acquainted; or marital adjustment; of the struggle of therapist and patient; of the formation of committees and organizations; of the socialization of children and adults in school, on the job, and in new communities; of occupational and professional rivalries; of intergroup contacts and conflicts; of the meetings of races and classes and nations.

The dynamics of one such struggle may be seen very clearly in Coleman's description of community conflicts.[8] The individual microprocesses of confirmation and disconfirmation produce their social counterparts in the form of cohesion and estrangement, alliance and enmity. Many of these conflicts begin around the attitudinal differences between separate groups—attitudes toward fluoridation, progressive education, unionization, the city manager plan, desegregation, communism in the schools, religious differences, and so on.

Community conflict typically begins with controversy around one or two specific issues and proceeds from there to include more general issues. A related transformation is for new and different issues to be brought into the dispute. The points of difference change from disagreements about issues to intense antagonisms between persons and groups, a shift that Coleman significantly describes as an attitude change.

As people seek out those who agree with them and cut their ties with those who disagree, the community tends to become polarized into two clusters. When social organizations do not exist in which people can find confirmation, new ones are created. At the same time, the pressure people exert on their associates to take their side results in existing community organizations being drawn into the controversy. New leaders emerge to take up the cudgels in the dispute; they are often people who have never before been in leadership positions. Informal meetings and word-of-mouth communications replace the formal channels of communication of the news media, which do not offer the kind of flexibility needed to carry on the struggle.

Derivation 1A

The greatest potential for mental disorder as well as for social conflict in a social group consists of deep, unresolved cleavages with respect to important attitudes (a) among the group members themselves, and (b) between the group members and members of other groups. It is in such groups that mutual and reciprocating disconfirmation is highest.

When a person is surrounded by others whose attitudes are similar or complementary, the feedback he receives from these others helps confirm his attitudes. To be like others in this sense and to feel confirmed in this way is to have a feeling of social solidarity with others, and to feel loved by them. To be like others is to find them pleasantly predictable, and thus to have a sense of stability, security, and order. To be like others is to be able to speak to them on their terms and thus to influence them (see Schachter, 27), and to be able to influence others is to have a sense of personal power. Love, security, and power are thus social products arising from social cohesion. From this standpoint, the definition of mental health in terms of the statistical norm has a certain utility and partial validity, although it is clearly inadequate from a conceptual viewpoint. In spite of all the criticisms of conformity that we have seen in recent years (most of them distorting the real issue, which is who is conforming to whom for what reasons and with what consequences), Homans' observation seems incontrovertible: the man without a group, *somewhere*, is a man who is in trouble.[13]

In disintegrated communities, we find lots of men who are in trouble. We may infer that disintegrated communities of the type described by Leighton and his colleagues are ones in which deep attitude cleavages are present.[14, 19, 20] Such communities have high frequencies of broken homes, few or weak associations between people, few patterns of recreation, a high frequency of hostility, crime, and delinquency, and a weak or fragmented network of communications. According to Leighton and his colleagues, more individuals were rated as "cases" in the disintegrated communities. "Indeed, our findings indicate that the level of integration of the community is more strongly related to mental health than is sex, age, or occupational position (20, p. 169)." Developing the lines of communication and the community organization needed to overcome disintegration and attitudinal cleavages would seem to be a natural task of preventive psychiatry.

It is not too speculative to infer that the high prevalence of mental illness among the lowest socioeconomic classes, as found in the New Haven and Midtown studies was due in part to the extreme disconfirmation experienced by people in these social classes.[12, 31] In America, the economic and social attitudes of the lower classes have not been very different from those of the rest of the population, particularly as regards the Horatio Alger myth that by hard work anyone can get ahead. This myth is tenaciously held in all sections of the population, but only in the lower classes is it persistently and powerfully disconfirmed. Not only do those of low status experience the disconfirmation of failure in a race in which everyone is somehow expected to win, but they are additionally stigmatized as characterologically deficient and rejected as personally undeserving of social respect. Srole (32, p. 360) calls this the "stigmatize-rejection" mechanism, and invokes it to help explain social class differences in the prevalence rates of mental illness. Snobbishness thus stands indicted as a pathogenic agent of mental illness, along with disintegration at the community level.

Derivation 2

Given enough time and freedom from outside influence, the struggles of individuals for confirmation in a social unit result in mutually equilibrating attitude changes that produce a stable social psychological structure, in other words, one that maximizes confirmation for all individuals.

Homans' dictum that "interaction produces liking" seems true enough as a statistical regularity, but it leaves out the mechanism by which this occurs.[13] For example, if I don't like you, and if we assume that you can't change, then the only way I can come to like you is to stop demanding and expecting things from you that you can't give me; I must change my attitude toward you. As I said before, liking is not an attitude, it is a by-product of an attitude that is confirmed. Interaction produces liking only through the medium of changed attitudes.

A stable social-psychological structure is not necessarily a healthy one. It is always healthy on its *own* terms, but it may not be healthy on *other* terms. A common constellation in a family, for example, is that if the parents are childish, the child assumes a parental role. These reciprocities are mutually confirming within the family. It is only when these attitudes are carried into social structures outside the family, usually by the child, that that family member experiences disconfirmation. The individual therapist working with a family member to change an attitude that defines a person's membership in an extremely important group faces a very tough job.

It is recognition of some such principal as *Derivation 2* to take the two most common examples, both involve bringing together all of the participants in a latent or overt conflict, inducing them to interact with each other, and then speeding up the process of mutually equilibrating attitude changes by means of therapeutic interventions. Only in Sartre's *No Exit* does a group of people, isolated from outside influences, remain locked in the hell of irreconcilable conflict for all eternity. In real life that is very unlikely.

With the advent of these social therapies, we are a long way from conceptions based on instinct liberation. The therapist, individual or social, must have a conception of how the attitudes of individual clients articulate with the norms of the numerous social systems through which they move, and of how the norms of these system mesh with each other and with larger and more inclusive systems. In a rapidly changing society that is deeply conflicted, the therapeutic options before us are extremely complex. Fitting a person to live in one group may unfit him to live in another while making a third group unfit for anyone to live in.

The newer social therapies, particularly those that deal with systems larger than the small group such as organizations and communities, also tend to blur the distinction between therapy and prevention.[22, 28] To produce an organization that has good communications and civilized means of conflict resolution involves changing the attitudes of the members in some highly therapeutic ways, sometimes as a condition of changing social practice, sometimes as a result of changing social practice. There is little difference between intervening in a social system to cure it and intervening in it to improve it. There is little difference psychologically between a therapeutic interpretation that reveals to an individual the true nature of his circumstances and a social analysis that shows men what they must do to save themselves. The words "therapy" and "prevention" seem inappropriate, somehow; "developmental social action*" may be worth thinking about.

CONCLUSION

The community mental health movement stands at the foothills of a practice that makes the heavy demands on theory I noted at the beginning of this paper—concern for both the normal and the abnormal, stability and change, the individual and the social, and prevention as well as therapy. This paper has presented the outlines of a concept that aims at fulfilling these needs, and has spun out some of its implications in rudimentary tests of its usefulness.

Attitude theory sees the driving force of man's activity as coming from himself, from his intentions, and from no external agency. The very shape of his mind, the sort of person he is, is the result of decisions he has made to alter some aspects of himself in pursuit of other aspects of himself. With every intended action man creates an infinity of novel activities and relationships, most of which are unintended and many of which contradict and disconfirm his intentions. Out of these disconfirmations come conflict, mental illness, individual and social change, new intentions, and sometimes learning and wisdom. Attitude theory is a theory of man entangling himself in the very bootstraps by which he hoists himself.

Although attitude theory attempts to be scientific rather than ethical, the beginnings of an ethical theory are in fact embedded in it, and this may increase its value to mental health workers. It is a fact that one of the most difficult attitudes to develop is a sense of responsibility, for one's self and for others. Just such a theory of responsibility lies at the heart of attitude theory. Our responsibility, individual and social, consists of the fact that everything that happens to us takes place with our participation, although not necessarily with our connivance. We are responsible for consequences of our actions that we do not intend as well as for those we do intend, since the former could not occur without the latter. It seems appropriate that a psychological theory of community mental health, if it does not begin with a statement of responsibility, should at least end with one.

REFERENCES

1. Arbuckle, D.S. Psychology, medicine and the human condition known as mental health. Community Ment. Health J., 2, 129-134, 1966.
2. Argyris, C. Interpersonal Competence and Organizational Effectiveness. Homewood, Ill., Dorsey Press, 1962.
3. Bellak, L., ed., Handbook of Community Psychiatry and Community Mental Health. New York, Grune & Stratton, Inc., 1964.
4. Benedict, R. Continuities and discontinuities in cultural conditioning. Psychiatry, 1, 161-67, 1938.
5. Boulding, K.E. The Image. Ann Arbor, Michigan, University of Michigan Press, 1956.
6. Brown, R. Models of attitude change. In R. Brown, E. Galanter, E.H. Hess, and G. Mandler, eds. New Directions in Psychology. New York, Holt, Rinehart & Winston, 1962.
7. Chein, I. The image of man. J. Soc. Issues, 18, 1-35, 1962.
8. Coleman, J. Community Conflict. Glencoe, Ill., The Free Press.
9. Deese, J.E. The Psychology of Learning. New York, McGraw-Hill Book Company, 1958.

10. Festinger, L.A. Theory of Cognitive Dissonance. New York, Harper & Row Publishers, 1957.
11. Heider, F. The Psychology of Interpersonal Relations. New York, John Wiley & Sons, Inc., 1958.
12. Hollingshead, A. deB., and Redlich, F.C. Social Class and Mental Illness: a Community Study. New York, John Wiley & Sons, Inc., 1958.
13. Homans, G.C. The Human Group. New York, Harcourt, Brace & World, 1950.
14. Hughes, C.C., Tremblay, M., Rapoport, R.N., and Leighton, A.H. People of Cove and Woodlot. New York, Basic Books, Inc., 1960.
15. Jacobson, E. Progressive Relaxation, 2nd. ed. Chicago, University of Chicago Press, 1938.
16. Kelly, G. The Psychology of Personal Constructs, New York, W.W. Norton & Company, Inc., 1953.
17. Lawrence, D.H., and Festinger, L. Deterrents and Reinforcements. Stanford, Calif., Stanford University Press, 1962.
18. Leeper, R.W., and Madison, P. Toward Understanding Human Personalities. New York, Appleton-Century-Crofts, 1959.
19. Leighton, A.H. My Name is Legion. New York, Basic Books, Inc., 1959.
20. Leighton, D.C., Leighton, A.H., and Armstrong, R.A. Community Psychiatry in a rural area. In L. Bellack, ed. Handbook of Community Psychiatry and Community Mental Health. New York, Grune & Stratton, Inc., 1964.
21. Malmo, R.B. Activation: a neurophysiological dimension. In R.J.C. Harper, C.C. Anderson, C.M. Christenson, and S.M. Hunka, eds. The Cognitive Processes: Readings. Englewood Cliffs, New Jersey, Prentice-Hall, Inc., 1964.
22. Nadler, E.B. Social therapy of a civil rights organization. J. Appl. Behav. Sci. (In Press).
23. The theory of the T. group and the theory of disconfirmation. Hum. Relat. Training News, 9, 5-6, 1965.
24. Osgood, C.E., and Tannenbaum, R.H. The principle of congruity in the prediction of attitude change. Psychol. Rev., 62, 42-55, 1955.
25. Phillips, E.L. Psychotherapy; A Modern Theory and Practice. Englewood Cliffs, New Jersey, Prentice-Hall, Inc., 1956.
26. Razran, G. The orienting reflex. In R.J.C. Harper, C.C. Anderson, C.M. Christenson, and S.M. Hunka, eds. The Cognitive Processes: Readings. Englewood Cliffs, New Jersey, Prentice-Hall, Inc., 1956.
27. Schachter, S. Deviation, rejection, and communication. J. Abnorm. Soc. Psychol., 46, 190-207, 1951.
28. Secord, P.F., and Backman, C.W. Personality theory and the problem of stability and change in individual behavior: an interpersonal approach. Psychol. Rev., 68, 21-32, 1961.
29. Schein, E., and Bennis, W., eds. Personal and Organizational Change Through Group Methods: The Laboratory Approach. New York, John Wiley & Sons, Inc., 1965.
30. Singer, E. Mind as Behavior and Studies in Empirical Idealism. Columbus, Ohio, R.G. Adams, 1924.
31. Srole, L., Langner, T.S., Michael, S.T., Opler, M.K., and Rennie, A.A.C. Mental Health in the Metropolis: The Midtown Manhattan Study. New York, McGraw-Hill Book Company, 1962.
32. Tomkins, S. Affect, Imagery, Consciousness. Vol. I, The Positive Affects. New York, Springer Publishing Co., Inc., 1962.

33. White, R.W. Motivation reconsidered: the concept of competence. Psychol. Rev., 66, 297-333, 1959.
34. Wolpe, J. Psychotherapy By Reciprocal Inhibition. Stanford, Calif., Stanford University Press, 1958.

Part Three
The Conference Model

THE CONFERENCE MODEL

This section of the book is devoted to a description of the conference model. It comprises a report of the events occurring before and during this American Nurses' Association first Community Mental Health Nursing Conference. Included are (1) a synopsis of the grant proposal including the rationale and objectives of the conference; (2) the work of the Advisory Committee in the selection of conferees and in the development of content, conference design, and the various forms used to facilitate the work of the conference (for example, glossary and evaluation forms); (3) the characteristics of the conferees, and those major themes, issues and recommendations which emerged during the course of the conference; (4) an analysis of the participants' evaluations of the conference; and (5) an annotated bibliography submitted by the conferees.

GRANT PROPOSAL

In order to obtain descriptive information about current nursing practice and innovative role activities in community mental health programs throughout the country, the executive committee of the ANA Psychiatric–Mental Health Division on Nursing Practice proposed a series of conferences to be held in three successive years (1970, 1971, and 1972). An application for a grant was submitted to the National Institute of Mental Health, Department of Health, Education, and Welfare of the United States Public Health Service. The first conference would be limited to invited registered nurses because of the urgent need for nurse colleagues to talk with one another about their work. The other two conferences were to be regional in nature and would include other mental health workers. (Funds have not been secured for these future conferences.)

RATIONALE

The proposal for the 1970 Conference included the following rationale:

1. . . . *in the last six years, nurses along with other health professionals employed in community mental health programs have been developing new ways to provide a variety of needed services to people and communities. Community mental health nurses indicated a need to describe their actual work experiences and to pool information with nursing colleagues, and report to the profession at large. Directors of graduate nursing programs and nurses in leadership positions in nursing service in the United States, as well as outside the country, continuously seek related information from ANA.*

2. *The proposed conference would assist in implementing a recommendation made in the 1967 Boston conferences "that efforts be made to encourage the development of widespread nursing interest in such programs."***

3. *Through the conference mechanism, the Division on Psychiatric and Mental Health Nursing Practice would provide opportunity to assist state nurses association Conference Groups on Psychiatric and Mental Health Nursing Practice to become viable mechanisms for the improvement of all aspects of psychiatric and mental health nursing service. The proceedings of the conference would help stimulate and encourage discussion and sharing of information among nurse members in SNAs which it was hoped would lead to greater interest and understanding, and the subsequent employment of nurses in a broad range of psychiatric-mental health facilities.*

4. *All professional nurses need to recognize the nature and sifnificance of the community mental health movement. They need to become involved in the issues and problems of health in a society in crisis. They need to enlarge the scope of their expertise regarding the total population of health care recipients. The clinical specialists in psychiatric nursing now employed in community mental health programs are in a unique position to influence others, particularly their nurse colleagues, in the planning and programing of community mental health services. This is one mechanism that could have impact for change in social institutions in the current social crisis.*

The conference was designed to re-emphasize the reciprocal relationship and interdependence between service and education. Community needs require an interdisciplinary approach and therefore nursing practice in community mental health programs has to be based on collaboration with other disciplines. Together with clients, the combined staff learn and test new practices to meet new needs.

The conferences emphasize: (1) those practices the nurse uses to focus on the immediate concerns of the clients, or on factors in the environment which elicit such concerns; and (2) those practices directed toward modification of

*"Short-term Clinical Training of Nurses for Community Mental Health Programs." Boston University, 1967.

these factors and toward strengthening existing institutions and resources which enhance self-actualization, and self-determination.

OBJECTIVES

The following objectives for the conference were proposed:
1. To bring together selected registered nurses currently employed in community mental health programs, for presentation and discussion of content describing selected nursing practices.
2. To obtain descriptions of nursing practices, concerns, and issues relating to innovation and expansion of role.
3. To publish the conference proceedings.
4. To disseminate this information—particularly to state conference groups on psychiatric nursing practice—as a recruitment tool for educational programs and for staffing community mental health programs, and to promote interest in conducting local conferences and workshops in order to improve community mental health nursing practice.

ADVISORY COMMITTEE

In June, 1969, the American Nurses' Association received notice of support for the first of three proposed conferences. With advice from the Executive Committee of the ANA Division on Psychiatric-Mental Health Nursing Practice, a five-member Advisory Committee was selected, all of whom were currently employed in community mental health programs. In July, 1969, Mrs. Elaine Goldman was named Project Director to coordinate the work of the Advisory Committee in the planning and implementation of the conference.

The Advisory Committee met for five days on two different occasions and concerned itself with the goals, format, content, and plans for evaluation of the conference and with the selection of the conferees. * To facilitate communication, a glossary was developed and distributed to the conferees. (see Appendix A).

Selection of Conferees

A list of 400 potential candidates was compiled by writing to a variety of sources such as community mental health centers, state nurses associations, psychiatric mental health conference groups, and graduate programs in

_____

* Dr. Herbert Butler, R.N., Nurse Consultant, Community Mental Health Centers Division, Mental Health Service Development Branch, National Institute of Mental Health, participated in the Advisory Committee meetings.

psychiatric-mental health nursing. In addition, information regarding the conference was publicized in nursing and medical journals, state nurses association bulletins, and selected newspapers.

The Advisory Committee developed criteria (see Appendix B) for the selection of 12 speakers and 50 participants for the conference.

The Advisory Committee, aware of the pressing need for community mental health nurses to describe and share information on practice, requested that nurse speakers "tell it like it is." Realizing the variation of roles developed in community mental health programs, the Advisory Committee planned that the conferees would represent the diversity in community mental health nursing practice and thus demonstrate that diversity itself is essential for creative responsiveness to a community's needs.

The Program

Four major topics, Community Involvement, Staff Development, Treatment Modalities, and Organization and Administration were selected by the Advisory Committee as a framework for presentation and discussion of content. For each of these four major topics, three speakers presented papers on relevant sub-topics.

    I. COMMUNITY INVOLVEMENT
       1. *"Community Mental Health in the City: Are They Really Patients?" Toni Francis, M.A., R.N.*
       2. *"The Role of the Nurse in Consultation and Education to Community Caretakers" Judith Anne Martois, M.S., R.N.*
       3. *"The Role for Nursing in a Community Drug Addiction Program" Judith Proctor, R.N.*

    II. STAFF DEVELOPMENT
       1. *"Differential Role Development for Nurses in Group Therapy" Janelle Ramsburg, M.S.W., R.N.*
       2. *"Emerging Issues in Training for Community Mental Health Nursing" Nancy French, M.S., R.N.*
       3. *"Implications for Nursing in the Training of Paraprofessional Workers in Community Mental Health Setting" Hilda Richards, Ed. M., R.N.*

    III. TREATMENT MODALITIES
       1. *"The Role of the Community Mental Health Nurse in a Rural Setting" Justina Neufeld, B.S., R.N.*
       2. *"Community Mental Health Nurses Question 'Care, Cure, and Coordination' " Margene Tower, M.S., R.N.*
       3. *"The Nurse Therapist as a Member of an Interdisciplinary Team" Sharon Gedan, M.S., R.N.*

    IV. ORGANIZATION and ADMINISTRATION
       1. *"Organizational Structure and Administrative Practice as They Affect the Nurse's Role" Norman Morse, M.A., R.N.*
       2. *"The Role of the Nurse in Development of Local Services*

Within a Statewide Mental Health Plan" Sarah Helen Carlton,
M.N., R.N.
3. *"The Nurse's Role In Planning Inner-City Mental Health Ser-*
   vices" Anita Narciso, M.S., R.N.

Each paper presented evolved out of the specific climate in which the nurse
functioned. Speakers described the community, the community mental health
program in which they worked and the responsiveness of the program to the
needs of the client. The discussion of the process of role development enhanced
their descriptions of their nursing roles.

Design of the Conference

The design of the three-day conference encouraged maximum participation
(see Appendix C). Conferees were divided and met as three heterogeneous
groups but convened as one group at the end of each day for summary reports
(see Appendix D). Throughout the first two days, conferees in each of the three
groups, meeting concurrently, heard and reacted to four presentations, one on
each of the four major topics. They examined and analyzed their own
experience in light of the speaker's conceptual framework.

THE CONFERENCE

The invited participants convened for three days in February, 1970, in New
York City, described the nature and scope of their nursing practice, and began to
clarify and conceptualize their operational frameworks. Major themes, issues,
problems, and questions evolved from intensive exploration and confrontation.
Some of these themes were general in nature and applicable to all mental health
workers; others were specific to the community mental health nurse.

Description of Conferees

The conferees came from 37 different states and the District of Columbia,
including inner-city, urban, suburban, rural and outreach areas. They spoke of
their nursing practice in, out of, and between psychiatric hospitals, and general
hospitals, health departments, community mental health centers, clinics and
satellite clinics, rehabilitation centers, institutions for the mentally retarded,
schools, churches, and related community agencies. An interesting phenomenon
was the variety of titles of the conferees. In the list of 12 speakers, there were no
two titles alike. Moreover, in the list of 50 participants there were 40 different,
though similar, titles.

Chief Nurse
Chief Nurse Therapist

Nurse Clinician
Clinical Specialist
Clinical Specialist Psychiatric Nursing
Nurse Specialist–Mental Health
Community Nurse Specialist
Community Mental Health Center Nurse
Mental Health Community Nurse
Mental Health Nurse
Mental Health Worker

The Content

The content of the conference will be summarized under the following headings:

1. *Composite View of the Community Mental Health Nurse*
2. *Educational Qualifications of Community Mental Health Nurses*
3. *Relationships with Paraprofessionals*
4. *Major Themes and Issues of Community Mental Health Nursing*

COMPOSITE VIEW OF THE COMMUNITY MENTAL HEALTH NURSE

The community mental health nurse was envisioned as a registered nurse, with a variety of educational and experiential backgrounds, who works in a setting within a community. Requirements call for mobility, flexibility, adaptability, and accessibility in responding to the needs of clients. By being a co-worker with the client, the community mental health nurse becomes more aware of her values and philosophy and must take into account the similarities and dissimilarities that exist between the client and the nurse.

Working with other members of the mental health team, the community mental health nurse may function in the following roles: therapist, liaison person, educator, consultant, supervisor, administrator, planner, community organizer, evaluator, and researcher. In addition to a sound background in the physical and social sciences, nurses in general and the community mental health nurse in particular, have refined their intuitive capabilities and sensitivity to stressful human experiences.

As a consequence, the community mental health nurse relates to disadvantaged clients in a more meaningful way than other professionals do. In many instances, nurses are the only professionals who work in all parts of the community.

Community mental health nurses described the preventive aspects of their role in mental health consultation with clients, particularly with caretakers such as public health nurses, teachers, religious, and formal and informal community leaders. Conferees told of their participation in social action within nursing, the mental health facility, and the community. They spoke of their involvement with, and commitment to, learning about people of diverse races and cultures. They agreed there is no quick and easy solution to problems related to the diversities of race and and culture. The conferees repeatedly stated that many current programs are irrelevant and "we would be better off without them." They agreed that what is really needed is social change, but opinions differed on the "how" and "rate" of change. Some pointed out that sudden changes induce anxiety, and result in behavior that provoke repercussions in the existing system; they feared the backlash of reactive repression which could give rise to greater evils; they hoped for real and lasting progress to come from collaborative processes that allow for true learning, trust, and consolidation of gains. Conferees described their programs and processes, based on different philosophies, but all aiming to promote mutual respect and to encourage self-determination and self-help.

Educational Qualifications of Community Mental Health Nurses

Possession of the appropriate credentials brings quicker recognition of the nurse's contribution and enhances her relationships with colleagues. At the present time nurses prepared as psychiatric-mental health clinical specialists at the master's level are scarce in many areas in the country and, undoubtedly, this situation will continue to exist.

Other nurses, less educationally qualified, need to be identified and prepared through continuing education and staff development programs to augment the services of the clinical specialist. How to prepare and utilize this nurse in the most efficient and economical manner evolved as one issue. Another issue that was discussed is whether or not nurses should use their skills to bring together and train groups of paraprofessionals in order to share the power and responsibilities included under the umbrella of nursing.

Relationships with Paraprofessionals

Several conferees described their understanding of nursing care, psychiatric nursing, education, and life. Several speakers described how their philosophy influenced their programs for training and utilization of the paraprofessionals. Participants spoke of their collaboration with paraprofessionals whose life experiences frequently enhance their relationship with consumers. There was general agreement that "learning is a two-way street."

Some of the speakers pointed out the necessity for anticipating needs and providing supportive services and opportunities for educational advancement and work mobility in order to insure a successful experience for the paraprofessional. They documented the fact that the paraprofessional is frequently the basic therapeutic staff member. A proposal was made to change educational systems so that they would accommodate and give due credence to the significant experience of individuals. There was consensus that the community mental health nurse must continue to broaden her practice and participate in a more meaningful way in bringing about social change in the community and in society in order to truly implement the proviso of "continuity of care."

MAJOR THEMES AND ISSUES OF COMMUNITY MENTAL HEALTH NURSING

Speakers identified changes, the processes of change, and the resistances to change in various nursing systems, including nursing education, nursing service, and the nurse herself. They indicated ways the community mental health nurse influences and is influenced by larger systems, that is, organized nursing, consumers, community mental health professionals and paraprofessionals, and community mental health institutions, communities, and society. While the official theme of the conference was change, the major issue was power versus powerlessness as related to the nurse's self-determination and accountability, and her ability in intiating and sustaining the process of change.

The issue of power was enmeshed in the need to shift from the "medical-model" to the "ecological-model" which allows for (1) the emergence of natural leadership based on the individual's competence and (2) an equitable shift of decision-making to all those concerned with the delivery of relevant services. There were divergent views of what this shift and the accompanying ideological struggle entail and, subsequently, the *essence* of the "ecological-model" emerged as a critical issue. Many conferees believed that sharing the power with other professionals, paraprofessionals, clients, and the community is the major concern—rather than the mere acquisition of power. This sharing of power is needed to bring about changes in systems that limit the mental health professional in dealing with the dysfunctional aspects of the community and society.

Conferees affirmed that additional and different kinds of personnel and methods of service are essential for the survival of community mental health nursing, which requires profound changes in philosophy, basic education, staff development, and continuing education programs. A recurrent theme of the conferees was the need for (1) a theoretical understanding of social systems, power and change, and (2) experiential learning in various human relations training programs, focusing on both group and individual phenomena and on the complex forces affecting the relationships between people.*

*For clarification of the similarities and differences between a variety of human relations training groups and group psychotherapy, see B. Lubin, and W. Eddy. The Laboratory Training Model: Rationale Method, and Some Thoughts for the Future. International Journal of Group Psychotherapy, Vol. XX, July 1970, No. 3. Reprints are available from Dr. Bernard Lubin, Division of Psychology, University of Missouri School of Medicine, 600 E. 22nd St., Kansas City, Mo. 64108.

RECOMMENDATIONS

The following recommendations for community mental health nursing emerged from the conference:

> Community mental health nurses have a responsibility to organize community mental health personnel in specific local and regional areas for interactional conference groups. Since no health discipline functions alone in the delivery of relevant health services, these regional conferences should bring together the consumers of service, paraprofessionals, and interdisciplinary professionals. The findings of this conference should be shared with the state and territorial nursing associations, and with the psychiatric-mental health nursing conference groups for consideration and action.

Conferees suggested that the nature and scope of community mental health nursing calls for a new definition of professionalism which, in turn, requires a new kind of education. Nurses need to develop a theoretical formula for the delivery of their services, based on a knowledge of social systems and theories of power and change.

The conferees stressed the need for nurses, together with paraprofessionals and other mental health professionals, to design learning experiences (such as interactional or personal awareness groups), or to use whatever means are available for increasing their abilities to understand, assess, and sustain people in periods of crisis. Out of the conferees' clinical experiences, postulates (see Foreword) and recommendations for action were derived. To validate these proposals, however, community mental health nurse practitioners and nurse educators should collaborate in designing and carrying through evaluative research regarding programs that involve the community mental health nurse.

Applied research projects should be instituted to identify: (1) community-based mental health problems; (2) elements of service which deal with community-based mental health problems; (3) the actual and potential contribution of various nursing personnel which may be (a) either professional or paraprofessional, or (b) others educated in different types of programs; (4) the contribution of various inservice and continuing educational experiences in nursing practice; and (5) evaluation tools for assessing the contribution to the mental health of people.

Findings from applied research should be used as content in the curriculums of various educational programs in community mental health nursing. In addition, these findings should provide guidelines for community mental health nursing practice, and should help in the development of standards for community-based mental health programs.

PROCESS

The structure of the conference was designed to maximize participation by all conferees in order to meet the objectives of the conference. Conferees were divided into three parallel sub-groups. Conferees had a wide range of experience and levels of authority in their own organizations. Characteristics of the sub-groups were established on the basis of the following: (a) designated leadership; (b) consistent membership; (c) spatial separation; (d) time limitations; and (e) predetermined primary tasks.

The content of the conference was embodied in four major areas from which 12 topics were selected for presentation. Each of the sub-groups heard and reacted to four different presentations during the first two days of the conference. On the third day, the nature of the assigned task changed and differed for each group. At the end of each day, the sub-groups combined to report their experiences.

It was apparent that the predetermined structure and content, the characteristics of the sub-groups, and the use of intergroup sessions provided the dynamics of the conference. The dynamics subsequently will be described in three phases; initial, interim, and closing.

The Initial Phase

The theme "change-agentry" and the issue of role relevance emerged early in the discussion of all the sub-groups relating the internal tasks of the conference to the external systems impinging on the conference; for example, the needs of the conferees versus the needs of community mental health nurses, or conference managers or clients. See diagram, top, page 225.

The topic of the power and authority of the Advisory Committee, the nursing profession, and institutions were interwoven in the discussion following the papers. While the presenters spoke to the theme of power and change, the subsequent discussions and processes expressed blocks to change that result in feelings of powerlessness. Conflict developed between group maintenance work and intellectual work, providing a struggle in the formation of work group relationships.

Conferees questioned their selection, risks involved in exposure, and expectations and limitations of the conference. There was concern over the format and structure, vocal and silent members, and an underlying conflict dependence versus independence. The group attempted to exercise its authority to change the prescribed structure and content but this never materialized. Some conferees felt "de-skilled" in the area of interpersonal competence because they were not able to use the status and power they had acquired in their agencies, and were compelled to re-establish themselves in a group of "chiefs."

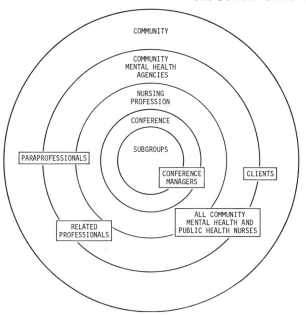

COMMUNITY

COMMUNITY
MENTAL HEALTH
AGENCIES

NURSING
PROFESSION

CONFERENCE

SUBGROUPS

PARAPROFESSIONALS

CONFERENCE
MANAGERS

CLIENTS

ALL COMMUNITY
MENTAL HEALTH AND
PUBLIC HEALTH NURSES

RELATED
PROFESSIONALS

Fig. 1.

The general mood of the initial phase of the conference was one of anxiety and frustration.

All three groups were confronted with problems related to designated and emerging leadership. The manner in which the three groups dealt with the role of leader and its accompanying authority helped determine the outcome, that is, the mastery of the task and the degree of satisfaction experienced at the conference.

The Interim Phase

This phase was exemplified by competition and conflict. There was evidence of competition in the group, between the groups, the community mental health nurses and other nurses, the other professionals, and the agencies represented. Conferees talked about experiencing personal conflict and group conflict. Dichotomizing and polarizing information and opinion emerged as a way of dealing with ambivalent feelings. The underlying theme appeared to be relative to a decision of a priority of "thinking" versus "feeling" or "getting on with the work while, at the same time, dealing with feelings."

As one conferee put it, "the study of process is not the task; process either facilitates or obstructs task performance." Clarification and restatement of the primary task followed. Discussion of the limitations imposed by the structure of the conference, directly attributable to conference management, served as a release for the conferees' feelings of anxiety and frustration. Conferees discussed the concept that community mental health nurses are less passive than nurses in general, and are more actively involved in risk-taking in order to bring about change. At the same time, conferees were actively seeking confirmation from their peers regarding these ideas. What resulted was the realization that community mental health nurses are functioning at different stages, in relation to their nursing practice and in their ability to articulate what they are doing.

In order to deal with emerging issues one group tried to "order" their conference experience, attempting to understand the phenomena of conceptualizing the conference via a model community—a community of peers and sub-communities with internal and external forces. The conferees seemed to recognize the need to coalesce in order to be productive. Work leaders emerged and common experiences, problems, and feelings were identified.

Closing Phase

In the final stage there was an attempt to reach closure and ascertain whether there could be a common understanding of the conference experience. This was reflected in the search for a common language (for example, "psychopolitics"), and a reconciliation of ideological and personal differences. Limitations of time, structure, and the heterogeniety of conferees prevented the accomplishment of these goals.

EVALUATION OF THE CONFERENCE IN TERMS OF CONFEREES' EXPECTATIONS*

The purpose of the evaluation is to determine the success of the conference in terms of meeting expectations of the conferees, and to assist future planners in identifying needs.

Method of Developing Evaluation Form

Prior to the conference, a questionnaire was mailed to all prospective participants, asking them to describe their expectations of the conference (see Appendix E). Based on an 85 percent return of questionnaires, the Advisory Committee developed a checklist of 15 expectations representing the varied needs of the conferees (see Appendix F). The check list was distributed four times at strategic points of the conference: before the conference, twice during the conference, and after the conference. Conferees were asked to rate each

---

* Reproduced by special permission of the publisher, National Training Laboratories, Institute for Applied Behavioral Science. Conference outcomes in terms of Participants' Expectations by D. Klein, *In* Urban Decision Making—The Findings From a Conference by Richard and Paula Franklin, 1967, Appendix B.

expectation as "high relevance," "low relevance," or "did not apply;" they were also asked to rate each expectation as "exceeded," "met," or "not met."

Method of Studying Responses

Analysis of the responses was limited to those conferees who returned all four evaluation forms. The data was summarized separately for each of the three work groups. In addition, an attempt was made to relate the extent to which the expectation was met to the degree of relevance that each particular expectation held for the conferee (see Appendix G). Other aspects considered were: (1) whether or not there were changes in relevance; and (2) the degree to which expectations were met.

SUMMARY OF FINDINGS

Responses to the checklist indicate which expectations were highly relevant for most conferees. They also suggest which of the highly relevant expectations the conferees felt were most satisfactorily achieved at the conference. In comparing the ratings of the three groups of conferees, relatively few differences were noted. In comparing the ratings of all conferees before, during, and after the conference, there was little change in what the conferees saw as relevant.

As indicated in Table 1, prior to the conference 50 percent or better of the conferees rate 12 of the 15 expectations items as having "high relevance." Apparently the composite checklist was a good representation of the opinions of the conferees. In comparing the pre-conference and post-conference ratings, there was little change in what conferees considered "high relevance." The exceptions were the three items listed below:

1. *Item 4: "to explore the impact of community mental health nursing on the profession" was rated "high relevance" by 62 percent of the conferees prior to the conference and by only 34 percent of the conferees after the conference. As was evidenced by some of the group discussion, community mental health nurses viewed themselves as a small group of nurses in a pioneering stage, struggling for survival. Consequently, they apparently could not address themselves to the important question of the impact of community mental health nursing on nursing as a whole.*
2. *Item 5: "to explore the impact of community mental health nursing on related disciplines" was rated "high relevance" by 67 percent of the conferees prior to the conference and by only 53 percent of the conferees after the conference. This may possibly reflect the fact that other disciplines were not present and this topic did not surface as a major concern. In the course of the conference, it seemed as though the energy of the group was consumed in role definition. However, many conferees asserted that members of related disciplines, and especially paraprofessions should be*

Table 1

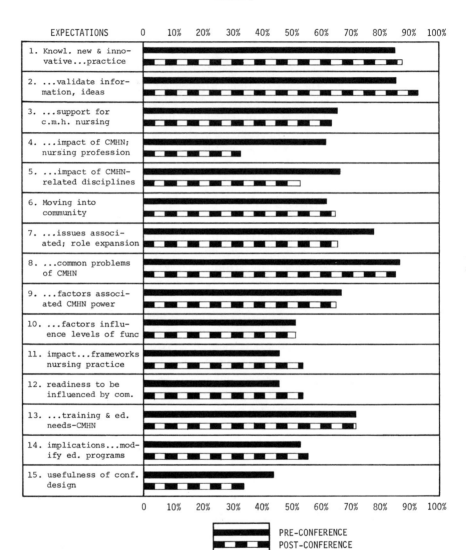

PRE-CONFERENCE
POST-CONFERENCE

included in future community mental health nursing conferences.
3. *Item 15: "to consider the usefulness of this conference design" was rated "high relevance" by 42 percent of the conferees prior to the conference, and by only 33 percent of the conferees after the conference. This item was proposed solely by the Advisory Committee and therefore did not necessarily reflect the expectations of the conferees.*

Since most of the items were considered to have "high relevance" by a

Table 2

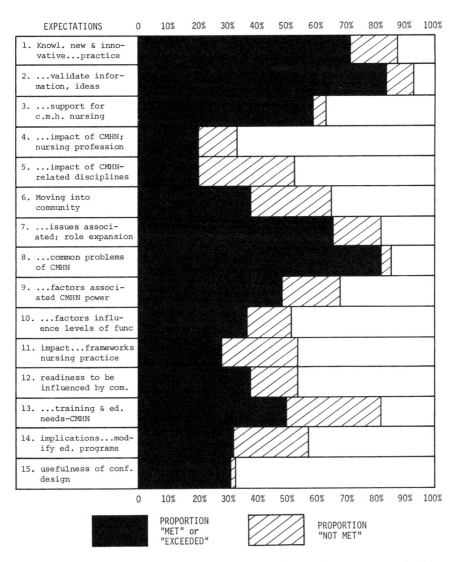

majority of conferees, an evaluation of the conference should report whether expectations were "met" or "exceeded." As an aid to future planning, it is important to identify the areas not met by this first national conference.

As indicated in Table 2, 13 out of 15 items were rated as "high relevance" by 50 percent or more of the conferees.

The following summary serves as an indication of the extent to which these relevant items were met:

Percent Met or Exceeded of those With High Relevance	Number of Items	Item No.
90-99	3	2, 3, 8
80-88	2	1, 7
70-77	3	9, 10, 12
60-66	2	6, 13
50-59	2	11, 14
40-49		
30-39	1	5

These figures would indicate that conferees felt the conference did not meet one item, (5) which had been considered to have "high relevance:"

> *Item 5: "To explore the impact of community mental health nursing on related disciplines" was rated "high relevance" by 53 percent of the conferees after the conference and, of the 53 percent, only 38 percent rated that the conference succeeded in meeting this expectation. Again, this item caused concern, which reinforces the need for future planners to include interdisciplinary participant and interdisciplinary content.*

On the positive side, eight of the "high relevance" expectations were considered to have been "met" or "exceeded" by 70 percent or more conferees. The conference was considered fairly successful in relation to the following eight expectations:

> *Item   8: "To identify common problem areas of nurses in Community Mental Health."*
>
> *Item   3: "To gain and provide stimulation and support for CMH nursing practice."*
>
> *Item   2: "To exchange and validate information and ideas."*
>
> *Item   1: "To gain knowledge of new and innovative forms of nursing practice."*
>
> *Item   7: "To explore issues associated with role expansion."*
>
> *Item 12: "To explore the nurse's readiness to be influenced by the community."*
>
> *Item 10: "To gain insight into the factors which influence levels of functioning."*
>
> *Item   9: "To understand the factors associated with the nurse's exercise of power in her setting."*

From the content of these eight items, it appears that:

1. Conferees responded to the opportunity to react to the presentations and to each other. Comments included: "there were no super-experts imposing their opinions on the group; people were on a peer level;" and "the variety of backgrounds and professional invovement provided an excellent oppor-

tunity to discover and explore in large and small groups, and individually in post-group encounters."

2. There was a general feeling of cohesiveness that developed from the conferees' genuine desire to share knowledge and experience in community mental health nursing. According to one conferee, the most important contribution was a clarification of what the underlying philosophy of community mental health nursing must be, and a better understanding of its role application.

3. Conferees successfully identified common problems without necessarily providing solutions.

There was concern regarding the structure of the conference. Some conferees believed that more than three days were needed to explore the evolving issues; others said that the groups were too large to permit optimum sharing of ideas. It is particularly noteworthy that according to Table 2, only 33 percent of the conferees rated Item 15, "To consider the usefulness of this conference design," as having "high relevance." However, of those conferees, 94 percent rated that the conference "met" or "exceeded" their expectations.

ANNOTATED BIBLIOGRAPHY

Beggs, L. Huckleberry's for Runaways. New York, Ballantine Books, 1969.
Written by the founder of the organization. Gives an account of its history. case experiences, and use of family therapy approach. Good insight into the problems of children who run away from home and implications for treatment.

Bindman, A.J., and Spiegel, A.D., eds. Perspectives in Community Mental Health. Chicago, Aldine Publishing Co., 1969.
A practical compendium of historical ideas and theories, contemporary viewpoints, and future prospects.

Clark, M. Health in the Mexican-American Culture: A Community Study. Berkeley, University of California Press, 1959.
Report of a research study giving excellent information about health practices and cultural behavior among Mexican-Americans.

Cowan, E., Gardiner, E., and Zax, M. Emergent Approaches to Mental Health Problems. New York, Appleton-Century-Crofts, 1967.
A series of excellent articles discussing innovative approaches to community mental health issues. Both philosophical and practical viewpoints are given.

Deloughery, G.W., Gebbie, K.M., and Neuman, B.M. Consultation and Community Organization in Community Mental Health Nursing. Baltimore, The Williams & Wilkins Company, 1971.
The authors develop the theory of mental health consultation and guidelines for practice. They cover the role of the nurse in community mental health planning, implementation and evaluation of services.

Duhl, L., and Leopold, R. Mental Health and Urban Social Policy. San Francisco, Jossey-Bass, Inc., Publishers, 1968.
Discussion of a variety of projects and programs both successful and unsuccessful. Helpful in looking at what made a failure as well as success of a program.

Evans, F.M.C. The Role of the Nurse in Community Mental Health. New York, The Macmillan Company, 1968.
A basic text beginning with a history of the development of community mental health and covering a wide range of new roles for nursing including a look at the international perspective.

Fagin, C.M. Family-Centered Nursing in Community Psychiatry-Treatment in the Home. Philadelphia, F.A. Davis, Co., 1970.
Graduate psychiatric nursing students describe their short-term psychotherapeutic endeavors in the home, followed by theoretical discussion by faculty members responsible for supervision.

Fuchs, L. Those Peculiar Americans. New York, Meredith Press, 1967.
". . . a scholarly yet personal and dramatic account of the tensions, conflicts, joys and changes experienced by the first 630 Peace Corp volunteers in the Philippines. . . ." An excellent discussion of the process of moving into a new situation and culture which is applicable to all professionals moving into new roles in community mental health.

Glasscote, R.M., and Gudeman, J.E. The Staff of the Mental Health Center—A Field Study. Washington, D.C., Joint Information Service of the American Psychiatric Association and the National Association for Mental Health, 1969.
Staff members in eight community mental health centers relate their work, worries, and hopes.

Grier, W.H., and Cobbs, P.M. Black Rage. New York, Basic Books, Inc., 1968.
Two black psychiatrists redefine mental health and illness in light of the history and current situation of the black race in this country.

Klein, D.C. Community Dynamics and Mental Health. New York, John Wiley & Sons, Inc., 1968.
Excellent presentation of how community dynamics affect programs and vice versa. Clearly delineates the elements and issues related to community mental health.

Kozol, J. Death at an Early Age. Boston, Houghton Mifflin Company, 1967.
The author describes his experience as a teacher in the Boston City Public Schools, revealing the subtle and not-so-subtle workings of a racist system.

Leininger, M. Community psychiatric nursing; trends, issues, and problems. Perspect. Psychiat. Care, VII:1,10-20, 1969.
Exploration of three major viewpoints regarding role expectations: the undifferentiated, differentiated, and ambivalent viewpoints.

Liebow, E. Tally's Corner. Boston, Little, Brown and Company, 1967.
An account of the Negro, street-corner society in Washington, D.C. One of the most insightful and moving descriptions of urban poverty and its effects among black males.

Lyford, J. The Airtight Cage. New York, Harper & Row, Publishers 1966.
A personal account of one man's fight with urban redevelopment in New York City. Also discusses in detail all the social systems and organizations as they relate to his environment.

Milio, N. 9226 Kercheval: The Storefront That Did Not Burn. Ann Arbor, The University of Michigan Press, 1970.
A public health nurse describes her feelings and impressions in relation to helping community people set up and operate a health care center in a lower southside ghetto in Detroit. The book points up that "those who would involve others, especially the poor, in the process of healthful change, must themselves be involved...."

Thomsen, M. Living Poor: A Peace Corps Chronicle. Seattle, University of Washington Press, 1969.
A personal account of a volunteer and his attempts to change-agent in a developing country. Discusses the many problems and the process that occurs.

Norman, J.C., ed. Medicine in the Ghetto. New York, Appleton-Century-Crofts, 1969.
A report of a conference which examined the health of ghetto dwellers. A recurrent theme was the extent to which racism can be blamed for the cause of the plight of ghetto residents.

McCormack, Sister Ann. The hospital is a community, too. Nurs. Outlook, 16:5,2-63, 1968.
Explores the various ways in which the psychiatric nurse may be of service to patients and staff of a general hospital.

Nylen, D., Mitchell, J.R., and Stout, A., eds. Handbook of Staff Development and Human Relations Training. Washington, D.C., National Training Laboratories, Institute for Applied Behavioral Science, 1967.
Provides useful ideas, information, and training activities relevant to a variety of situations and cultures.

Parad, H.J. ed. Crisis Intervention: Selected Readings New York, Family Service Association of America, 1965.
Excellent basic text for theory of crisis intervention.

Shore, M.F. and Mannino, F.V., eds. Mental Health and the Community: Problems, Programs, and Strategies. New York, Behavioral Publications, 1969.
Focuses on the struggles of translating community mental health ideas into specific action programs.

Stokes, G.A., ed. The Roles of Psychiatric Nurses in Community Mental Health Practice: A Giant Step. Maimonides Medical Center—Community Mental Health Center, 1969.

An explanation of the processes by which the extended roles of psychiatric nurses in a specific community mental health center setting were developed and institutionalized.

Storlie, F. Nursing and the Social Conscience. New York, Appleton-Century-Crofts, 1970.

Nurses and nursing organizations are indicted and challenged to act on the "real issues"—the injustices of society which both produce and maintain poverty and ill health.

Ujhely, G.B. Determinants of the Nurse-Patient Relationship. New York, Springer Publishing Co., Inc., 1968.

A valuable framework for thinking and acting that makes it easier for the nurse to apply the principles of nurse-patient relationships to any specific situation.

GLOSSARY

I. *CONCERNS* — a matter for consideration; marked interest or regard usually arising through a personal tie or relationship*

II. *ISSUE* — a matter that is in dispute between two or more parties; a point of debate or controversy*

III. *COMMUNITY* — one concept of community is the population within the geographic boundaries. Another concept of community deals with a membership based on a community of interests, and/or a psychologic sense of belonging together. These may be manifested in ethnic, religious, socio-economic or other groupings.

IV. *COMMUNITY MENTAL HEALTH PROGRAM* — is one which envolves from and is responsive to the community need. It is a collaborative effort between the professions and the community which plans, develops, delivers, and evaluates services.

V. *ROLE* — is a pattern of expected behaviors which is brought about by the interaction of the self and others within a given social system.

VI. *NURSING ROLE IN COMMUNITY MENTAL HEALTH PROGRAMS* — is a combination of expected and evolving patterns of behavior related to her concept of nursing and those of her peers, the perception of clients (individual and communities) and related disciplines.

*Webster's Seventh New Collegiate Dictionary

APPENDIX B

CRITERIA

Speakers must meet following criteria:
a. Experience: minimum of two years practice in community mental health programs.
b. Education:
    1. Post-graduate training programs in community mental health nursing;
    2. doctoral and master's degrees in psychiatric-mental health—community mental health nursing;
    3. baccalaureate degree, AA, and diploma graduate in nursing with inservice education in community mental health programs.
Participants must meet one of the following criteria:
a. Practitioners in community mental health programs.
b. Faculty of graduate psychiatric-mental health programs, teaching and supervising students in community mental health programs.
c. Graduate students involved in above.
d. Consultants

APPENDIX C

A.N.A. CONFERENCE ON COMMUNITY MENTAL HEALTH NURSING
FEBRUARY 25-27, 1970
THE AMERICANA HOTEL, NEW YORK, N.Y.

WEDNESDAY

9 am	Versailles Terrace	
	WELCOME	
	PLANS FOR CONFERENCE	
Chelsea A	Chelsea B	Buckingham A
I	II	III
Speaker 1	Speaker 2	Speaker 3
DISCUSSION	DISCUSSION	DISCUSSION
10 am		
11 am	BREAK	
I	II	III
Speaker 4	Speaker 5	Speaker 6
DISCUSSION	DISCUSSION	DISCUSSION
12:15	LUNCH	

THURSDAY

9am Chelsea A	Chelsea B	Buckingham A
I	II	III
Speaker 7	Speaker 8	Speaker 9
DISCUSSION	DISCUSSION	DISCUSSION
10 am	BREAK	
10:15		
Speaker 10	Speaker 11	Speaker 12
DISCUSSION	DISCUSSION	DISCUSSION
11:15		
I	II	III
THEMES	THEMES	THEMES
12:15	LUNCH	

FRIDAY

9 am Chelsea A	Chelsea B	Buckingham A
WORK SESSION:	WORK SESSION:	WORK SESSION:
CONFERENCE REPORT	*CONFERENCE EVALUATION*	*CONFERENCE APPLICATION*
Input	Input	Input
Discussion	Discussion	Discussion
10:30	BREAK	
11 am		
WORK SESSION: DISCUSSION	WORK SESSION: DISCUSSION	WORK SESSION: DISCUSSION
12 Noon	LUNCH	

1:15

WORK SESSION: SUMMARY REPORT TO CONFERENCE	WORK SESSION: SUMMARY REPORT TO CONFERENCE	WORK SESSION: SUMMARY REPORT TO CONFERENCE

3 pm

Versailles Terrace

REPORT FROM THREE GROUPS

4 pm

1:30

I SUMMARY REPORT TO TOTAL CONFERENCE	II SUMMARY REPORT TO TOTAL CONFERENCE	III SUMMARY REPORT TO TOTAL CONFERENCE

3 pm — BREAK

3:30

Versailles Terrace

REPORT FROM THREE GROUPS DISCUSSION

5 pm

5:30-7 pm

PRINCESS BALLROOM
DUTCH TREAT COCKTAIL PARTY

APPENDIX D

THE 1970 CONFERENCE ON COMMUNITY
MENTAL HEALTH NURSING

Group I	Group II	Group III
Eva Anderson	Gertrude Johannsen	Ellen Andruzzi
Cherryl Blakeway	Lois Batton	Joye Bradley
Elizabeth Carter	Esther Bigelow	Herbert Butler, *Recorder*
Rose Marie Davidites	Mary Cantrell	Frances Carbone
Fernando Duran	Sarah Carlton, Speaker	Alice Clarke
Nancy Fasano	Linda Copeland	Sharon Gedan, Speaker
Toni Francis, Speaker	Barbara Davis	Margaret Hardin
Priscilla Gretsch	Richard Drake	Lydia Hill
Mary Henderson	Rhetaugh Dumas	Janice Hitchcock
A. Naomi Kennedy	Nancy French, Speaker	Evelyn Kennedy
Sister Sheila Lyne	Cathleen Getty	Linda Laws
C. Elizabeth Madore, *Recorder*	Marie Groth	Nancy Mayes
Winifred Maher	Catherine Harris	Donna Miller
Sandra Matteson	Sharon Janzen	Mary Ann Muranko
Ruth Miller	Margaret Johnson	Sister Ann McCormack
Norman Morse, Speaker	Ruth Lewis, *Leader*	Anita Narciso, Speaker
Evelyn McElroy	Judith Martois, Speaker	Dorothy Nayer
Justina Neufeld, Speaker	Judith Moore	Jeannette Nehren
Phyllis Parnes	Mabel Morris	Cornelius Neufeld
Janelle Ramsburg, Speaker	Norma Schapera	Elizabeth Patterson
Alice Robinson	Ruth Seigler, *Recorder*	Judith Proctor, Speaker
Rachel Robinson, *Leader*	Barbara Teague	Hilda Richards, Speaker
Kathryn Schlichtmann	Frank Tosiello	Janice Ruffin, *Leader*
Anita Stoddard	Margene Tower, Speaker	Jonna Smith
Kathryn Wheeler	Phyllis Wentz	Frances Williams
Concha Yenoukian		Rothlyn Zahourek

APPENDIX E

A goal of the ANA Conference on Community Mental Health Nursing is to represent the ideas, aspirations and needs of its planners and participants. The Advisory Committee will prepare an evaluation procedure for this conference and asks for your cooperation. *Please list specific outcomes which, if achieved at the conference, would make it a success for you.* e.g., gain knowledge of new and innovative forms of nursing practice.

It will facilitate the work of the committee if you will please type or print on this page and return it by February 13, 1970. These pre-conference expectations will be compiled by the committee for the use of all conferees.

Signed   Date

APPENDIX F

1970 COMMUNITY MENTAL HEALTH NURSING CONFERENCE
Evaluation Form #4

Name: _____

Group: _____

INSTRUCTIONS: For each of the expectations listed below, please indicate (with an X) the relevance that each item has for you at this time and whether it was "exceeded," "met," or "not met" during the conference.

Expectation	High Rele-vance	Low Rele-vance	Does Not Apply	Exceeded	Met	Not Met
1. To gain knowledge of new and innovative forms of nursing practice.						
2. To exchange and validate information and ideas.						
3. To gain and provide stimulation and support for C.M.H. nursing practice.						
4. To explore the impact of C.M.H. nursing on the nursing profession.						
5. To explore the impact of C.M.H. nursing on the related disciplines.						
6. To explore ways of moving nurses into the community.						
7. To explore issues associated with role expansion.						
8. To identify common problem areas of nurses in C.M.H.						
9. To understand the factors associated with the nurse's exercise of power in her setting.						
10. To gain insight into the factors which influence levels of functioning.						
11. To study the impact of theoretical and ideological frameworks on the practice of nursing.						
12. To explore the nurses' readiness to be influenced by the community.						
13. To gain knowledge of training and educational needs for C.M.H. nursing practice.						
14. To explore the implications for modifying basic and graduate programs.						
15. To consider the usefulness of this conference design.						

APPENDIX G

RATINGS OF CONFEREES (N-54) ON EXPECTATIONS: HIGH, LOW, OR NO RELEVANCE

CHECK LIST #

Expectation	High Relevance				Low Relevance				Did Not Apply
	Exceeded Expecta- tion	Met Expecta- pectation	Did Not Meet Ex- sponse	No Re- sponse	Total High Rele- vance	Exceeded Expecta- tion	Met Expecta- tion	Did Not Meet Ex- pectation	No Re- sponse	Total Low Rele- vance
1. Knowledge new & innovative ... practice									
2. ...validate informa- tion, ideas									
3. ...support for C.M.H. nursing									
4. ...impact of CMHN; nursing profession									
5. ...impact of CMHN related disciplines									
6. Moving into community									
7. ... issues associated: role expansion									
8. ...common prob- lems of CMHN									

APPENDIX G (Continued)

Expectation	High Relevance					Low Relevance					
	Exceeded Expectation	Met Expectation	Did Not Meet Expectation	No Response	Total High Relevance	Exceeded Expectation	Met Expectation	Did Not Meet Expectation	No Response	Total Low Relevance	Did Not Apply
9. ...factors associated CMHN power											
10. ...factors influence levels of function											
11. impact ...frameworks nursing practice											
12. readiness to be influenced by community											
13. ...training & educational needs – CMHN											
14. implications ...modify educational programs											
15. usefulness of conference design											

Form used to tabulate " G " – data –